Hormone Harmony
Over 35

A New, Natural Whole-Body Approach
to Limitless Female Health

By Dr. Michelle Sands, ND

Free Hormone Healing Bonuses and Video Content

I know you are busy, so I created a simple video series, cheat sheets and additional tools to give you the key takeaways, plus some extra resources to help you fast-track to living your limitless life!

Go here:

https://glownaturalwellness.com/hormoneharmony

ISBN 13: 9781726602303

Kindle Direct Publishing, a DBA of Amazon Services LLC

Seattle, WA

Edition 1.0.1

Free and Frequent Updates!

'm frequently updating this book with the latest research, resources and

information based on the feedback you share and developments in endocrine and epigenetic science.

If you are reading this book on a Kindle or Kindle App, make sure it's the latest version.

To get the latest and greatest, just open your app, click or press the "More" icon in the lower right-hand corner and then press "Sync" and you'll always be up to date. See the image below.

To my incredible husband, my best friend, Jeff:
You've helped me to follow my passion, realize my dreams and create an
amazing life. You're my hero.

And my son, Paxton:
You amplify my gratitude for being alive
and you have been the inspiration for my research and life's work.

I love both of you so much.
You are my universe.

My family and friends: you have all played a significant role in shaping my
life's experience and who I am today. And for that I am forever grateful.

Coach Shea:
Thank you for believing in me and showing me how to believe in myself. Your
simple advice has become my mantra: "Your body can do anything you want it
to, all you need to do is feed it, train it and believe in it."

To my amazing practice members—
Thank you for entrusting me with your most valuable asset and allowing me
to serve you.

Disclaimer

I want to help you not only balance your hormones, but leverage your genetics with the power of nature so that you can heal, balance and thrive. Having said that, although I am a doctor, I am NOT YOUR doctor (Unless, of course, I am). The information in this book is based on my years of clinical experience, personal history, research, and education. However, all statements should be viewed as my opinions.

The contents of this book, associated websites, videos, apps, and documents are for educational purposes and should in no way be construed as medical advice.

I have included references in the back of the book for those who would like to seek more information.

Please seek medical supervision before attempting to do anything recommended or alluded to in this book. If there's a tiebreaker to be made, don't listen to me. Trust your instincts. Bottom Line: Don't do anything stupid with your or someone else's life.

Table of Contents

A Note to You, the Reader

"The real secret to life-long good health:
Let your body take care of you."

- Deepak Chopra

Hi! I am Dr. Michelle Sands, ND, a Naturopathic physician with a passion to help women take charge of their health and happiness naturally. I am not an author by trade, but a physician. But I am writing this book because I believe the messages, ideas, tools and resources provided within these pages can truly change your life.

There is nothing that I want more for you than to give you hope even when you think there is none to receive. I spent the better part of my early adult life believing that I was broken, that my hormones stopped working, and that there was nothing that could be done by me.

I believed that because I kept hearing that message over and over again. Doctor after doctor, specialist after specialist, all offered prescriptions, but no solutions. However, something deep within me, or perhaps far bigger than me, told me there was more to it than I realized. I was not going to find answers at the bottom of a child-safe prescription bottle. Instead, something told me to seek real answers. Something told me I shouldn't accept a Band Aid solution and then lose hope, so I dug deep and took my health into my own hands.

You see, *that* is what I want for you. I want to empower you so you can take *your* health into your own hands.

If you picked up this book, chances are you're struggling with some aspect of your health. And you likely know, or at least suspect, that your struggles have something (if not everything) to do with your hormones.

Maybe you recently found out you have a hormonal imbalance. It could be that you've known it in your heart for a while, but just haven't been able to get the help you need or find the answers that will bring your health back.

Perhaps you've been taking hormone replacement therapy or birth control pills for years, but they just aren't cutting it. Maybe you've heard that there is a better path to healing, one that would allow you to feel better.

Most likely, you're reading this due to a growing list of confusing symptoms with possible origins in hormone imbalance. These include experiencing hair loss, anxiety, weight gain, joint pain, mood issues, extreme fatigue, allergies, sexual dysfunction and brain fog. The list really goes on and on, but you get the picture.

Whatever your story, I feel for you and I'm here to help. I've had my own struggles with PMS, depression, fatigue, joint pain, and infertility, that went on for decades. I was chasing the diagnosis, but not looking at the big picture.

I was frustrated with the lack of answers and lack of support from the conventional medicine community. I knew deep down that the answer wasn't in another pill. And I know what it's like to feel like you have to figure everything out on your own.

It wasn't until I applied a more holistic way of looking at hormone imbalances and used a systems-based approach that I was able to finally uncover the real reasons for my hormonal imbalances.

It took years of research and testing, using myself as a guinea pig, then later working with hundreds of women, before I was able to produce a proven protocol for hormone balance and healing. Eventually, I went on to help thousands of other women do the same with this protocol.

Despite what so many doctors told me for over 10 years, I gave birth to my wonderful son, Paxton. And I did it all naturally.

The sad reality is that hormone imbalances and insufficiencies are now more common than ever. Plus, with the average lifespan extending well past the age of menopause, women are faced with many more years of suffering and struggle.

To make matters worse, it's unfortunate that the conventional medical system we've learned to rely upon only serves to leave us worse off. Women are often misdiagnosed, or even worse, dismissed by their primary care providers.

So wherever you are in your healing journey, no matter how badly you feel, or how many doctors you have seen -even if you've been told that there is no hope- I want you to know that things *can* get better and *will* get better as long as you commit to taking charge of your own health and make the changes to get your life back.

Buying this book is an excellent first step. And I'm so happy you picked it up because I'm honored to be part of your journey.

Introduction

Our hormones naturally start to decline around the age of 30. In a perfect world, this slow, gradual, graceful decline would gently take you into menopause and beyond, with everything staying in perfect harmony.

For the majority of us, we fall far short of this perfect world. Our hormones are less like the Philharmonic Symphony and more like a tone-deaf high school garage band. And the decline feels more like a punch in the face.

Have you noticed that you are waking up more tired than you were when you went to bed? Are you noticing weight gain and extra flab on your arms and belly despite no change to your eating habits and regular workouts? Are you experiencing a slowdown of your mental function, lapses in memory and ability to focus? Do you feel like you are aging faster than you should?

The New "Normal"

I see women every day through my virtual practice who are frustrated with who they have become. They explain to me that they feel as if they are trapped in someone else's body. They often feel like they aren't even in control of theirs brains.

Concerned, they make an appointment with their primary care doctor. And if they are lucky, he will agree to run some blood tests. More often than not, those tests come back "normal". The doctor kindly lets them know that "nothing is wrong."

Unfortunately, pressing the issue with most doctors will land you a prescription for sleeping pills and antidepressants, but not real answers. (Later, when I share my story, you will see how this exact thing happened to me.)

How in the world can "nothing be wrong"? Is it normal to feel tired and moody all of the time? Is it normal to not be able to get a good night's sleep and to not have any desire for sex? Is it normal to gain fat and lose muscle and bone? The answer, in my opinion, is NO! Not at all. These women do not feel fine, so something must be wrong. The reason conventional medicine can't provide answers is because it isn't a disease or condition that can be billed to insurance.

Here is a news flash. **The absence of a diagnosed disease or health condition does NOT equal Wellness.**

Wellness is an active process of becoming aware of and making choices toward a healthy and fulfilling life. Wellness is more than being free from illness. It is a dynamic process of change and growth. It is...

"...a state of complete physical, mental, and social well-being, and not merely the absence of disease or infirmity."

- The World Health Organization

...a conscious, self-directed and evolving process of achieving full potential."

- The National Wellness Institute

Maintaining an optimal level of wellness is absolutely crucial to living a higher quality life. Wellness matters. Wellness matters because everything we do, every emotion we feel, relates to our well-being. In turn, our well-being directly affects our actions and emotions. It's an ongoing circle. Therefore, it is important for everyone to achieve optimal wellness in order to subdue stress, reduce the risk of illness and ensure positive interactions.

And for women over 35, a major component in optimizing wellness is hormone balance.

Why are Our Hormones so Out of Tune?

Life is very different today than it was just a few decades ago. As women, we have more opportunities and responsibilities. And we are exposed to more toxins and stressors than our mothers and grandmothers ever were.

Don't get me wrong, I am all about progress, modern conveniences, higher education and equal rights. But all of these come with a price.

Raising a family, managing a household, and excelling in a career adds a lot of extra responsibility and pressure on our bodies *and our hormones.*

Sure, hormone decline while aging is a completely natural process that our mothers, grandmothers and women before them experienced, long before we were toting a briefcase in one hand and a diaper bag in the other.

However, in the last 30 years, studies have shown that female hormone levels are dropping earlier and faster than ever before. In fact, recent research has determined that today's women are experiencing a 30-50 percent drop in hormones between the ages of twenty and forty. Twenty and Forty! What this means is that the symptoms that we typically used to associate with aging women are now being experienced by women as young as 25. This new "normal" is not okay.

This rapid decline of hormones isn't solely due to increased responsibilities and the do-it-all mentality we have all adopted. Accelerated hormone decline is compounded by environmental stressors.

For example, toxins in our environment are like kryptonite for our hormones. Every moment of our lives we are exposed to thousands of toxic substances. They enter our bodies with each breath, meal or drink we take, the clothes and cosmetics we wear, the things we encounter every day in our homes, workplaces and while traveling.

The innocent looking cleaning supplies under your sink, your favorite lotion in that pretty bottle, pesticides on the healthy fruits and vegetables you eat, chemicals in your plastic water bottle, and the round-up sprayed on your neighbor's lawn are all known hormone disruptors, or xenobiotics. Ongoing exposure to these hormone disrupting toxins will do a number on your hormones. The sad truth is we are seeing these effects on younger and younger women, with more and more teens than ever struggling with hormone imbalances.

Don't worry, I'm not proposing that you quit your job, stay inside your home and hold your breath. This book isn't about creating fear and scarcity, since there is enough of that out in the world already. What you will learn in this book will help you improve your health while living the most exciting, vibrant life possible.

In the pages that follow, I will show you two very important things:

1. I will show you the ways to reduce the number and frequency of stressors your body is exposed to (mental/emotional, physical, chemical, and spiritual)

2. I will show you how to leverage your genetics to optimize your wellness, making you more resilient to the stressors that cannot be avoided

We will look at what hormones are, what they do, how they get out of balance and why a whole-body approach is absolutely necessary for true and lasting hormonal balance.

Have you ever asked yourself: Why is it that so many women are on Hormone Replacement Therapy (HRT) and STILL feel like crap? How can this be possible? If hormones are low, and we give our body hormones, shouldn't we get where we want to go?

I know this will break your heart to hear, but the answer is no. It isn't that simple. If it were, I wouldn't need to write this book and you wouldn't need to read it. Instead we'd all be laying on a beach somewhere in our Victoria Secret bikini, hanging out with Oprah and Beyoncé, being waited on by our hunky husbands, while we close million-dollar business deals from our cell phones and congratulate our oldest children on their Nobel Peace Prizes.

Okay, balanced hormones won't exactly look like that. But life does get a whole lot easier and rose-colored when your hormones are in harmony.

So why is it that taking hormones doesn't fix the problem?

Here is the truth that many health practitioners will not tell you, especially the ones prescribing your hormones:

Hormone Harmony is about so much more than having the right *amount* of hormones in your body. It is also about FUNCTION: whether or not those hormones are able to effectively show up for work on time, perform their jobs and then clock out. This will all make more sense later, but ultimately, we have to optimize not only the production of hormones, but also the function of hormones and the organs they are communicating with in order to truly feel well.

This means a whole-body approach.

What Are Hormones?

Even with the popularity of hormone therapies, most women really don't understand what hormones are and how they work. It is only when problems start popping up in our late 30's and beyond (sooner for some of us) that we give our precious hormones any real attention.

Hormones are our body's communication system. They are chemical messengers that deliver information to our cells, turning on and off processes to regulate or control many of our bodily functions.

When hormones are in balance, it is like a beautiful symphony with all of its various instruments playing their individual part and coming together melodiously in tune. However, if one instrument plays off key, it can ruin the harmony and disrupt the entire symphony.

This is what happens when we have imbalances and deficiencies in our hormones. Too much or too little of one hormone will impact all of the others over time. These imbalances can impact your sleep, mood, weight, hair, skin, nails, energy level, sex life, brain function and even your happiness.

For optimal wellness, your hormones must be balanced and in harmony.

When I say the word hormone, what comes to mind for many women are the BIG THREE sex hormones: Estrogen, Progesterone and Testosterone. These hormones are extremely important for your health and well-being, and we will be talking about these in-depth later in this book.

However, in order to balance these hormones, we must also address the other hormones that are so important to our health and well-being, which include:

- Cortisol
- Insulin
- Glucagon
- Leptin
- Ghrelin
- Thyroxine
- DHEA
- Pregnenolone
- Human Growth Hormone
- Melatonin
- Neurotransmitters
- Vitamin D (Yes, this is actually a PRO
- Hormone)

We will dig into many of these hormones and what you need to know so you can take control of your body and your life and make your hormones work for you.

Welcome to Hormone Harmony
Over 35

T his book is for you if you want the very best out of life. It's for you if somewhere along the way you lost your edge. Maybe you aren't as sharp, fast, strong or witty as you used to be. Maybe you've lost your libido, your energy, or even your passion for life. However, you know that there should be - that there is - so much more that you could be experiencing and so much more joy you could be feeling, and you aren't willing to settle for just feeling "Okay", much less feeling bad or depressed.

My goal for is simple: to help you or someone you care about navigate the confusing world of hormones and thrive.

My aim is to simplify the confusing journey, so you'll experience a lot less pain, hardship, confusion and the overwhelm that *I and so many women like you have endured.*

Th is book will help you save time and simplify the experience, making getting your life back clear and painless, with the fewest number of complications and side effects as possible while maintaining (if not improving) your most significant relationships. In fact, I feel completely comfortable promising that you will emerge from this experience a better person than when you began.

If you have a short attention span, brain fog, or you learn better and faster with videos, then go to:
https://glownaturalwellness.com/hormoneharmony
where you can watch my Hormone Healing Made Simple series, take additional assess-ments and download some great resources and bonus content to help you reach your goals.

xix

Here's what to expect, along with an additional bonus video, so you can get the most out of what I'm going to tell you in the shortest period of time.

First, it's interactive. There are lots of opportunities for you to go deeper into the content and gain access to the free videos, resources, and other tools that I've provided. You can even reach out to my private women's only community and connect with other women like you.

Second, this book is intended to help optimize health, with no BS. I have no hidden agenda. My only incentive is to share my experience to ensure you live your best life.

Third, it's for people who want to live life to the fullest and are interested in living optimally, no matter what it takes. I take on controversial points of view in this book, and at times may push your belief systems. I'm not here to make you comfortable or to be your best friend. I'm only interested in results. In other words, I'm not on anyone's side, I'm not controlled by special interests or insurance companies. I'm not driven by the fear of lawsuits and I'm not motivated by money. I'm passionate about wellness, that's it. That is the side I'm on. So, if you already have a preconceived notion of what you think is right or wrong in terms of health, healing or hormone balance, then you might as well close this book right now. But before you decide to close this book, ask yourself: How good do you really feel? How truly happy are you? If you've spent your life listening to conventional medicine and something still doesn't feel right, it may be time to open your ears and listen to what I have to say.

Now, if you don't want BS, and do want simple truth from a heart-centered physician who, not too long ago, felt hopeless when it came to her own hormone struggles, then please read on. This book explains the truth, not insurance company approved junk nor pharmaceutical industry funded crap. The strategies and tools in this book have helped thousands of women to heal, balance and thrive so that they can have children, build families, run companies, create art, and find the joy that makes life worth living.

Finally, this book is packed with easy to understand concepts, easy-to-implement recommendations and lots of great ideas. I

don't just want you sitting around reading what I have to say, I also want you taking action and optimizing your wellness.

My intention is to give you hope, to inspire you, motivate you, and give you needed clarity, focus and knowledge, so you can make good decisions without feeling as though you have to second guess yourself throughout a complex process that often results in frustration and even more symptoms.

How to Use this Book

've divided the book into 3 sections.

*　*　*

Section 1 - Section 1 gets you acquainted with the endocrine system, including the major organs, and introduces you to the main hormones and their functions, symptoms of imbalances, and quick tips to improve the function of each hormones. This section also includes self-tests that give you an idea of which of your hormones might be out of balance. You'll also get some great resources, such as which tests to ask your doctor for, and optimal blood test ranges. Plus, I'll share my favorite way to test hormones - no blood required.

*　*　*

Section 2 - In Section 2 we will cover what it is that turns good hormones bad, as well as endocrine disruptors and how to avoid them. I share the story of how my devastating hormone diagnosis at age 20 paved the way for thousands of women to achieve real balance.

You'll learn why my infertility and hormone imbalances didn't improve with hormone treatments, no matter how many I tried. I'll outline my philosophy on healing through a holistic, systems-based approach to hormone balance that honors the interconnectedness of every body system and the bio individuality of every woman. And I'll explain why this works every... single... time.

*　*　*

Section 3 – In Section 3 I give you a true jumpstart to hormone balance and focuses on the diet and lifestyle practices to improve detoxification, digestive health, blood sugar balance, eliminating endocrine disruptors and reducing stress along with restorative practices to promote natural hormone balance.

This final section is less about reading and all about doing. My goal for every reader of this book isn't just to have you walk away with more knowledge. I want you to walk away in better condition - physically, mentally, and spiritually - than you were before.

I have included my complete *21 Days to Hormone Harmony Program,* which is all in here for you to implement. I've included meal plans, recipes, shopping lists, daily protocol sheets and everything you need for support.

The majority of women who complete this 21-day program report a massive increase in energy, better digestion, more restful sleep, an average weight loss of 8-10 lbs, and a healthier relationship with food and themselves.

One Quick Tip

Reading this book is a big win for you. I applaud you for that. Getting to this page; the fact that you are reading these words tells me you have an even greater chance of success. However, it is only those who implement the strategies I outline that will truly see results. Despite the popular saying, Knowledge is NOT Power. Inspired action based on knowledge is what truly equals power.

If you want to skip all the reading and just jump into Part 3, you can begin getting results right away.

So, GO FOR IT! You have my blessing. My feelings won't be hurt if you don't read the book cover to cover. The truth is, there is nothing I want more for you than for you to feel amazing. So, flip through, take the assessments in section one, read about the imbalances that came up on your assessment, jump into the 21-day plan, and be sure to reach out to me and let me know how you are doing. The *21 Days to Hormone Harmony Plan* in Section 3 is complete on its own, so you can start there and read the rest of the book while you are healing.

I'd absolutely, positively, love to hear from you, to get to know you better, and have you share your success story, your transformation, a before and after picture of yourself or a video, and comment in my private women's only Facebook group, <u>The GLOW Tribe</u>:

https://www.facebook.com/groups/218880138852353

Virtual Hugs,
Dr. Michelle

P.S. I wrote and edited this book with the help of a couple special people (mostly my husband) in a very short time. There are absolutely, positively some spelling, grammatical, and layout errors. It was more important for me to get the message in as many women's hands as quickly as possible than it was for me to get perfect punctuation.

If you happen find one (or more) mistake, please do me a favor, and send an email to support@glownaturalmedicine.com. Note the page number, sentence, and mistake and I'll fix it right away. Thank you for your help in advance.

I'm all about results, implementation, and speed, and I've chosen to give you a resource that will help change your life, rather than attempt perfect grammar.

P.P.S. If you love this book or you've found it helps you or someone you care about, will you please post a review on Amazon. Nothing will make me happier than to hear your personal transformation, and each review helps other women find the book, so they too can benefit.

P.P.P.S. If you don't like this book, please just send me an email and tell me why. I will gladly give you your money back. Please be kind. My intentions in writing this book are to help you.

Hormone Harmony Self-Assessment

Let's go ahead and start with the most important thing: YOU. I want you to start by thinking about which hormones you want to focus on and which ones you feel are fine on their own.

This self-assessment is a good starting point, but it isn't accurate. With that said, you can get pretty far in healing your own hormones armed with just the information I'm about to tell you. However, since many hormone symptoms overlap, you may wish to get more definitive numbers from some of the testing I recommend in the next section. This will help you to confirm the results of your assessment.

Before you begin the 21-Day Program at the back of this book, I recommend taking this short hormone self-assessment to understand where your current imbalances are. At the end of the program, and again six weeks later, I recommend answering the questions again. This will help you track your symptom changes, stay on top of any new issues, and help you troubleshoot the next steps to hormone harmony.

Give yourself ONE (1) point for each item that applies.

Section 1

____ Are you constantly racing from one task to the next?

____ Do you feel wired yet tired?

____ Do you struggle to calm down before bedtime?

____ Difficulty falling asleep or disrupted sleep?

____ Do you worry about things beyond your control?

____ Are you quick to jump to judgment and feel offended?

__ Do you have poor memory or feel distracted, especially under duress?

__ Sugar cravings (You need "a little something" after each meal)?

____ Bone loss (Do you have a diagnosis of osteopenia or osteoporosis)?

__ High blood pressure or rapid heartbeat?

____ High blood sugar?

____ Indigestion?

____ More difficulty recovering from physical injury than in the past?

__ Irregular menstrual cycles?

Section 2

__ Fatigue or burnout?

__ Loss of stamina, particularly in the afternoon from two to five?

__ A negative way of thinking?

__ Decreased ability to concentrate?

____ Feeling stressed most of the week?

____ Insomnia or difficulty staying asleep?

____ Low blood pressure (not always a good thing, since your blood pressure determines the correct amount of oxygen to send through your body, especially into your brain)?

____ Postural hypotension (You stand up from lying down and feel dizzy)?

____ Do you catch every cold that comes into town?

__ Asthma? Bronchitis? Chronic cough? Allergies?

____ Low or unstable blood sugar?

____ Salt cravings?

__\ Excess sweating?

___ Muscle weakness, especially around the knee?

__\ Muscle or joint pain?

Section 3

__\ PMS or PMDD?

___ Cyclical headaches (particularly menstrual or hormonal migraines)?

___ Painful and/or swollen breasts?

___ Irregular menstrual cycles or cycles becoming more frequent as you age?

__\ Heavy or painful periods?

__\ Bloating, particularly in the ankles and belly, and/or fluid retention?

___ Ovarian cysts, breast cysts, or endometrial cysts (polyps)?

___ Easily disrupted sleep?

__\ Itchy or restless legs, especially at night?

___ Miscarriage in the first trimester?

Section 4

__\ Bloating, puffiness or water retention?

___ Abnormal Pap smears?

__\ Heavy bleeding or postmenopausal bleeding?

___ Rapid weight gain, particularly in the hips and butt?

___ Tender breasts?

___ Fibroids?

_____ Endometriosis or painful periods? (Endometriosis is when pieces of the uterine lining grow outside of the uterine cavity, such as on the ovaries or bowel, and cause painful movements.)

_____ Mood swings, PMS, depression, or just irritability?

_____ Weepiness, sometimes over the most ridiculous things?

_____ Mini breakdowns? Anxiety?

_____ Migraines or other headaches?

_____ Insomnia?

_____ Brain fog?

_____ A red flush on your face (or a diagnosis of rosacea)?

Section 5

_____ Poor memory?

_____ Depression, perhaps with anxiety or lethargy that lasts more than two weeks?

_____ Premature wrinkling?

_____ Night sweats or hot flashes?

_____ Trouble sleeping, waking up in the middle of the night?

_____ A leaky or overactive bladder?

_____ Bladder infections?

_____ Droopy breasts?

_____ Achy joints?

_____ Minimal interest in exercise?

_____ Bone loss as diagnosed by a DEXA test?

_____ Vaginal dryness, irritation, itchiness down there?

_____ Dry eyes, or just dry skin?

___ Low libido?

___ Painful sex?

Section 6

___ Constant craving for sweets?

___ Inability to go more than 3 hours without food?

___ Feeling like you need "a little something" after dinner?

___ Get irritable without sugar or bread?

___ You get shaky when you are hungry?

___ Have a waist circumference of more than 35" (89cm)?

Section 7

___ Trouble losing fat?

___ Have you lost muscle tone?

___ Is your hair falling out, tangled and dry?

___ Are you nails breaking easily?

___ Do you take longer to recover from workouts than you used to?

___ Are you noticing increased wrinkles and loss of skin elasticity?

___ Do you experience joint pain?

Section 8

___ Do you feel sluggish?

___ Muscle weakness?

___ Fatigue?

___ Sleep disturbances?

___ Reduced sex drive?

___ Decreased sexual satisfaction?

___ Do you experience weight gain?

___ Fertility issues?

___ Irregular menstrual cycles?

___ Vaginal dryness?

___ Loss of bone density?

Section 9

___ Do you experience abnormal hair growth on my face, chest, abdomen?

___ Acne?

___ Oily skin and/or hair?

___ Areas of darker skin (e.g. armpits)?

___ Thinning hair on your head and hair that tangles easily?

___ Skin tags?

___ Depression and/or anxiety?

___ Have PCOS?

___ Difficulty getting pregnant (trying for 6+ months)?

Section 10

___ I have brain fog or feel like my memory isn't quite what it used to be.

___ I'm losing hair (scalp, body, outer 3rd of my eyebrow).

___ My hair tangles easily.

___ I feel constipated often and need a stimulant (like caffeine) to get a movement.

___ I'm frequently cold and/or have cold hands and feet.

___ My periods are sporadic or greater than 35 days apart.

___ Joint or muscle pain.

___ Dry skin.

___ Difficulty getting pregnant (trying for 6+ months) or have had a first trimester miscarriage.

___ Low mood or depression.

___ I'm tired, no matter how much I sleep.

___ Don't sweat as easily or as often.

What Your Results Mean....

Give yourself a point for each Yes answer. The higher you score in a section, the higher the probability you have the corresponding imbalance. At least 3 points in a section indicates that there is likely an imbalance

5 Section 1 = You may have high cortisol

7 Section 2 = You may have low cortisol

4 Section 3 = You may have low progesterone

6 Section 4 = You may have estrogen dominance

6 Section 5 = You may have low estrogen

4 Section 6 = You may have insulin resistance or pre-insulin resistance

1 Section 7 = You may have Low Growth Hormone

5 Section 8 = You may have Low Testosterone

4 Section 9 = You may have Too much Testosterone

5 Section 10 = You may have Low Thyroid

Section I

CHAPTER 1

Before The Pause

E astern cultures call it, "A Woman's Second Spring".
Westerners refer to it as "The Change"!

Most women in my circles just refer to it as, "Hell".

Pretty much every woman over 35 is familiar with menopause. And, at least in Western cultures, pretty much every woman over 40 fears it, some worse than death itself.

The wrinkles, the pot-belly, saggy skin, crepe-y legs, dried up vagina and brain fog aren't things that anyone is looking forward to. Western societies view menopause as "the end of the line" or "the expiration date" on our feminine appeal.

For Eastern cultures, the view of aging is very different for both men and women. Rather than nearing an ending, menopause is looked at as a new beginning, as a woman's "second spring". It's a time of renewal and a passing to a wiser, more respected and cherished status in the community.

Menopause Around the World

Menopause, defined by the World Health Organization, is the permanent cessation of menstruation, and marks the end of a woman's reproductive years. As a biological event for women around the world, menopause itself is universal. However, research shows that the symptoms and cultural significance of menopause are not.

In the United States, women (and the media) associate menopause with symptoms such as hot flashes and night sweats.

Surprisingly, these complaints are not universal. In fact, the main symptoms of menopause vary among cultures. In 1970, Marcha Flint, an anthropologist, first attempted to look at the menopausal experiences of women in non-Western cultures. She studied 483 women in India and found that most didn't complain of symptoms during menopause, other than menstrual changes. A decade later, Margaret Lock found that the symptom most likely to be reported by Japanese women during menopause was shoulder stiffness, while hot flashes were actually very rare.

In a Hong Kong study, researchers found that joint and muscle problems were the most common symptoms. In all of these studies women reported symptoms as "mild."

What could be the reason for these very different physical experiences of menopause?

Current research suggests that lifestyle may play a bigger role than previously thought. Another idea is that the most important factor determining a woman's experience of menopause is the culture in which she finds herself before, during, and after menopause. In our youth-idolizing Western culture, menopause can seem like an ending. However, in many cultures, menopause is a time of new respect and freedom for women. A study reported that Mayan women, although experiencing some uncomfortable symptoms, looked forward to menopause, as it provided newfound freedom and status. Marcha Flint's study in India found that women who were veiled and secluded before menopause could now go to the same places that men socialized and drink beer while having fun.

Regardless, I believe that all women, no matter their background, health history or prior belief systems, can use the tools I outline in this book to make menopause and peri-menopause a time of energized freedom.

Before the Pause

Do you remember that awkward transition period when you were just becoming a teenager? Your body started doing weird things you didn't understand. Your brain started behaving in ways you couldn't control. Puberty was a confusing time for us as young girls, but at least some of us had the support of a mother that let us know what was happening, that it was normal, and that we were not going crazy or dying of some rare infectious disease.

Perimenopause is a similarly awkward time for women in their thirties and forties. It kind of sneaks up on us and we often don't even know it's happening. In fact, many women, and some doctors, don't even really understand what Peri-menopause is. There is no other time in a woman's life (other than puberty) associated with so many significant physical and emotional changes. Unfortunately, unless your physician has been educated on anti-aging and functional medicine, they'll likely miss or even dismiss this very real problem. The reason being is because most MD's are trained to diagnose and treat disease rather than how to create and optimize wellness.

You see, perimenopause and the hormonal imbalances associated with it is NOT a disease. However, it can really mess with your quality and enjoyment of life.

Now, let's talk about what perimenopause really is:

Perimenopause: It's the lovely period right before our ovaries shrivel up for good and resemble nothing but a pair of dried raisins attached to our ever-thinning uterus.

I kid, sort of.

Seriously though, what the heck is Perimenopause? Let's dissect the word.

According to my Google dictionary, the word "Peri" reveals:

pe·ri

□pirē/

noun

noun: **peri**; plural noun: **peris**

(in Persian mythology) a mythical superhuman being, originally represented as evil but subsequently as a good or graceful genie or fairy.

peri-

prefix

prefix: **peri-**

around; about.

The "peri" we are talking about here is the latter, the prefix meaning "around or about". However, I couldn't help but notice that the first definition is also pretty spot on - maybe those Persian Mythology geeks were actually women in their 40's.

Perimenopause is that ambiguous timeframe somewhere after age 30, when a woman is still cycling, and everything seems to be rolling along fine, but suddenly the wheels start falling off.

Now, this isn't the case for everyone, but the more I look around, the more I see wheels by the side of the road, while two and three wheeled buggies clunk along in a futile effort, trying to keep the pace they are used to.

Going through this change will look different for every woman, since some do manage to sail through it with flat tummies, stable moods, and a vibrant glow. If that is you, congratulations. Perhaps you lived a very healthy and wholesome lifestyle, thus managing to avoid endocrine disrupting toxins, pharmaceuticals, junk food and stress. Or maybe you are one of the genetically gifted and resilient lucky few that never really had to think about health yet managed to stay thin and blemish free her entire life. Either way, congrats.

Now, if you're like the rest of us, the other 99.8 percent of women in the western world, you are likely experiencing some pretty troubling symptoms.

Let me ask you, did your hourglass figure suddenly morph into something closely resembling SpongeBob Square Pants?

Would you rather read about sex than actually have sex with your spouse?

Do you often misplace your keys, wallet or glasses?

Are you less confident, expressive or outgoing than you used to be?

Are you experiencing depression, anxiety, trouble sleeping, headaches, joint pain, bone loss, muscle aches…?

You get the picture. Chances are, if you have one or more of these symptoms, your hormones are out of harmony.

The challenge is trying to boost specific hormones while also trying to precisely recalibrate others in order to restore balance and harmony.

In the chapters that follow, I will show you how to balance your own hormones and optimize your overall wellness using lifestyle strategies such as nutrition, exercise and movement, rest and recovery, stress reduction, mindset and meditation, and supplementation.

But first, it's important to understand a little more about where your hormones come from and what they do.

CHAPTER 2

Your Hormone Factory

"If I have to draw attention away from some hormone induced acne on my chin, I wear a lot of mascara"

—Oliva Wild

You might say endocrine glands are the boss-babes of the body: They tell your cells what to do and when to do it. Without your endocrine glands (and the hormones they release) your cells wouldn't know when to do the important things that make your body function. Without your hormones, you would die.

The endocrine system is a series of glands that produce and secrete hormones that the body uses for a wide range of functions. These control many different bodily functions, including:

- Respiration
- Metabolism
- Reproduction
- Sensory perception
- Movement
- Sexual development
- Growth
- But where do hormones come from?

Hormones are produced by glands and then sent into the bloodstream to the various tissues in the body. They send signals to those tissues to tell

7

them what they are supposed to do. When the glands do not produce the right amount of hormones, dysfunction and disease can develop and affect many aspects of life.

Your Neuro-Endocrine Organs

The Hypothalamus: This gland runs the show. The hypothalamus is located in the brain and controls the pituitary gland, which releases the following types of hormones:

Thyrotrophic-releasing hormones, which signal the pituitary to produce Thyroid Stimulating Hormone (which goes on to tell the thyroid to make thyroxine).

Growth-releasing hormones, which stimulates the pituitary to produce Human Growth Hormone.

Corticotrophin-releasing hormones, which stimulate the pituitary to release ACTH, which in turn stimulates the adrenals to make cortisol.

Gonadotropin-releasing hormones, which signals the pituitary gland to send hormonal messages to the ovaries in women and testis in men.

These hormones start the intricate communication and biofeedback system that ultimately regulates most of the body's control systems such as temperature, appetite and weight, mood, sex drive, sleep and thirst.

The Pituitary Gland: This gland is often referred to as the "master gland" of the body. The pituitary gland is the first in the chain of command from the hypothalamus. It greatly influences all of your organs and its function is vital to your overall wellbeing. The pituitary gland has two parts, the front and the back, each producing different hormones.

The front of the pituitary gland, commonly called the anterior pituitary, produces the following types of hormones:

Growth hormone (HGH): This hormone promotes growth in childhood. For adults, it helps to maintain healthy muscle and bone mass, aids in healing and recovery, and its loss is often associated with the signs of aging. We will discuss this hormone in more detail later.

8

Prolactin: In women, it stimulates milk production. Overproduction can lead to PMS and painful cramps. In males, low levels are linked to sexual problems.

Adrenocorticotropic (ACTH): I nearly never call this hormone by its name, but rather its initials. Its job is to tell the adrenal glands to produce cortisol, the "stress hormone." This is very important because many times when people are told their adrenals aren't functioning, it is really a lack of ACTH that is the cause rather than the adrenals themselves.

Thyroid-stimulating hormone (TSH): Just as the name implies, this hormone helps to regulate the body's thyroid, which is crucial in maintaining a healthy metabolism. This hormone is often measured to assess thyroid function. However, since it is a pituitary hormone, it tells us little about the actual function of the thyroid gland.

Luteinizing hormone (LH): In women, this hormone regulates estrogen. In men, it regulates testosterone.

Follicle-stimulating hormone (FSH): Found in both men and women, it stimulates the release of eggs in women and helps ensure the normal function of sperm production in men.

The back part of the pituitary gland is called the posterior pituitary. It produces the following two hormones:

Oxytocin: This hormone causes pregnant women to start having contractions at the appropriate time and also promotes milk flow in nursing mothers. This is the love hormone that gets secreted when we give and receive hugs or other skin-to-skin contact.

Antidiuretic hormone: Commonly referred to as vasopressin, this hormone helps to regulate water balance in the body.

The Pineal Gland: This gland is shaped like a pinecone (from where it gets its name). It's responsible for the production of melatonin, the hormone that helps us fall asleep. The pineal gland is greatly influenced by light and dark.

The Parathyroid Gland: This gland produces parathyroid hormone, which is vital to proper bone development. It helps control both calcium and phosphorus levels in the body. The parathyroid gland is actually a group of four small glands located behind the thyroid gland.

The Thyroid: This is a butterfly-shaped gland in the front of the neck that controls your metabolism.

The thyroid gland secretes hormones that govern many of the functions in your body, such as the way the body uses energy, consumes oxygen and produces heat. Thyroid disorders typically occur when this gland releases too many or too few hormones and are quite common in women over the age of 35. An overactive or underactive thyroid can lead to a wide range of health problems.

Unfortunately, most conventional MD's are taught to only measure TSH, which is a pituitary hormone and they fail to measure any of the action markers of thyroid function such as T3, T4, RT3, and T3 Uptake, which -more often than not- causes MD's to miss and dismiss thyroid dysfunction in many women (Check out the "Tests to Ask Your Doctor For" section in this book to be sure your doc is running a full thyroid panel).

The Thymus: You don't hear much about this gland, but it does have an important function. This gland secretes hormones that are often referred to as humoral factors. The role of these hormones is to make sure a person develops a healthy immune system.

The Adrenal Glands: These are a pair of walnut sized glands that sit atop the kidneys and produce the hormones for stress, namely, adrenaline and cortisol, but also produce androgens including DHEA and a little bit of women's testosterone. As we enter into perimenopause and menopause, we women do lean on our adrenal glands tremendously to pick up the slack as our ovarian production declines. For this reason, we're going to focus a great deal more on the adrenals later in this book.

The Pancreas: The main function of the pancreas is to maintain healthy blood sugar levels. It is a large gland located behind the stomach that produces insulin, glucagon, and other hormones.

Diabetes occurs when the pancreas does not produce enough insulin or when the body doesn't use insulin properly.

The Ovaries: These glands produce eggs and sex hormones, including estrogen, testosterone, and progesterone, which are vital to reproductive organ development, breast development, bone health, pregnancy, fertility, sex drive, mental focus, mood and body composition.

Three Systems in One

The Neuroendocrine system is really a collective of three major systems in the body, with the hypothalamus and pituitary gland in control. These systems integrate the nervous and the endocrine system together:

HPA Axis - Hypothalamic - Pituitary - Adrenal

HPT Axis - Hypothalamic - Pituitary - Thyroid

HPG Axis - Hypothalamic - Pituitary - Gonadal (Ovary)

These systems are not really separate, but they all interact with each other. And it's never just about topping off a hormone, since if you're low in progesterone and hoping that you can just take some progesterone and call it a day, that isn't really how hormone balancing works. The supplemental hormone may help you initially, but you really have to look at thyroid health and adrenal health and even beyond that to find what is causing the low progesterone in the first place.

Your Own Personal "Philhormonic"

Remember how I said that in many ways your hormones are similar to a large symphony, like a philharmonic? Or should we say "Philhormonic"? There are many different sections like the strings and the wind and percussion, each with its individual instruments and unique musicians. When the curtain rises, all of the many instruments and sections come together in perfect harmony, each playing its own individual part within the harmony.

Our hormones must balance and work in concert with each other in order for us to look and feel well. They have to know their jobs, but also be alert of changes in pace, production or functionality of each other and then adjust accordingly. In perimenopause and menopause, too little or too much of one hormone will set off a domino effect, causing imbalances in other hormones throughout the system.

11

I see this in my practice all of the time. Whether it's Jessica, the busy homeschool mom who makes all her family's meals from scratch and bikes with her children each day, who at age 38 started experiencing horrible menstrual cramps, migraines and mood swings for the first time in her life. Or Denise, the interior designer who suddenly began snapping at her colleagues, vendors and spouse. "I'm really hard to be around lately," she told me. Or Cyndi, a successful bank executive who suddenly began to lose her edge at work, having trouble concentrating, taking longer to perform tasks and feeling absolutely exhausted at the end of her workday. "I used to go to spin class after work and still have fuel in the tank. I don't know how that has happened".

These three women came to me with very different symptoms. They all led very different lives in different cities. All three had previously seen their primary care physicians and were told not to worry, that what they were experiencing was normal; that it's because they are stressed, because they have kids, because they have jobs, because they work too many hours, workout too hard, don't work out at all, eat too much, eat too little …etc.

Let's take a quick look at the symptoms these three women were complaining of:

- PMS
- Cramping before and during menses
- Migraine Headaches
- Mood Swings
- Temper
- Loss of Patience and Reasoning
- Fatigue
- Brain Fog

These are all classic symptoms of hormonal imbalance. However, neither the women nor their doctors made the connection to perimenopause, likely because hot flashes and night sweats (the symptoms most commonly associated with menopause) were not an issue they were having.

The problem for all three women was the decline in one or more hormones that started a chain reaction in their body, ~~which ended up~~ presenting a wide variety of symptoms. The good news is all three women were able to regain their balance naturally without prescriptions or medical intervention.

Here's the deal: perimenopause and menopause are very natural states and seasons in a woman's life. However, because of modern stresses and toxicities, the natural states of hormonal decline are happening sooner and more abruptly than our bodies can handle, and this is what leads to these unfavorable symptoms.

As you enter perimenopause, hormone production declines significantly in the ovaries, and the adrenal glands need to pitch in and make up the difference. When menstruation ceases and we enter menopause, the ovaries stop producing hormones altogether. Our bodies are designed to handle this decline in hormone production by calling in the adrenals as a backup to help us maintain our quality of life. Sounds perfect, right?

So then what is going on? Why are these women experiencing symptoms? Well, our adrenals just aren't able to keep up with the demand of our modern lifestyle. By the time we hit perimenopause, we've already taxed our adrenals beyond their ability and we are left with insufficiencies and imbalances that extend far beyond the endocrine system into immunity, detox, digestion and energy production.

CHAPTER 3:

The Symphony Players: Your Sex Hormones

"I believe that love and forgiveness engages an incomprehensible healing force and sometimes true healing occurs, but always an emotional and spiritual healing happens."

–Angeli Maun Akey

efore we get into assessing your hormone balance, let's talk a little bit about each hormone to give you a better understanding. You can skim through this section and read about the hormones that are of interest to you or skip ahead to the Hormone Self-Assessment, then come back and look at the hormones that were most impacted on your assessment.

The Steroid Hormones

Steroid hormones are derived from cholesterol and are lipid-soluble molecules. Examples of steroid hormones include the sex hormones (androgens, estrogens, and progesterone) and hormones of the adrenal glands (aldosterone, cortisol, and androgens).

Steroid hormones cause changes within a cell by first passing through the cell membrane of the target cell. Steroid hormones, unlike non-steroid hormones, can do this because they are fat-soluble. Cell membranes are composed of a phospholipid bilayer (read "layer of fat"), which prevents fat-insoluble molecules from diffusing into the cell.

14

Steroid Hormones do their job in the following way:

Step 1: Steroid hormones pass through the cell membrane of the target cell.

Step 2: The steroid hormone binds with a specific receptor inside the cell.

Step 3: The receptor bound steroid hormone travels into the nucleus and binds to another specific receptor on the chromatin.

Step 4: The steroid hormone-receptor complex calls for the production of messenger RNA (mRNA) molecules, which code for the production of proteins, which builds muscle and allows for important functions in the body.

Types of Steroid Hormones

Adrenal Gland Hormones

Aldosterone: This mineralocorticoid acts on the kidneys promoting the absorption of sodium and water. Aldosterone aids in blood pressure regulation by raising blood volume and blood pressure.

Cortisol: This glucocorticoid aids in metabolism regulation by stimulating the production of glucose from non-carbohydrate sources in the liver. Cortisol is also an important anti-inflammatory substance and helps the body deal with stress. We will be discussing cortisol in more detail later.

Sex Hormones: The adrenal glands produce small amounts of the male sex hormone testosterone and the female sex hormone estrogen. This is key for women as they head into menopause, as we depend on healthy adrenal glands to produce sex hormones when our ovaries retire.

Gonadal Hormones

Testosterone: This is often thought of as a male sex hormone, however, it is very important to female health, as we will discuss later.

Estrogen: These female sex hormones are produced in the ovaries. They promote development of female sex characteristics, skeletal growth and so much more.

15

Progesterone: This female sex hormone is produced in the ovaries and important for the production and maintenance of the uterine lining during pregnancy. This is also what I like to refer to as Nature's Valium, since it is our calming hormone.

Now, let's examine some of these hormones in a bit more detail.

The Big Three: Your Sex Hormones

Estrogen

Estrogen is one of the three main sex hormones that women have. Another name for these hormones is steroid hormones. I know, it sounds like something you pick up at the male locker room at Golds Gym. But in this context, the word steroid simply means that the hormones are made from cholesterol. The other main steroid is progesterone and testosterone. Estrogen is responsible for female physical features (like breasts and hips) and reproduction. Men have estrogen too, but in smaller amounts.

Why is estrogen important?

Estrogen helps bring about the physical changes that turn a girl into a woman. These changes include:

- Growth of the breasts
- Growth of pubic and underarm hair
- Start of menstrual cycles
- Estrogen helps control the menstrual cycle and is important for child-bearing

Estrogen also has other functions that you may not be aware of:

- Keeps cholesterol in control
- Protects bone health for both women and men
- Affects your brain (including mood), bones, heart, skin, and other tissues

You can see from these other functions why hormone health is important to whole-body health and how disturbances anywhere might throw off the delicate balance.

Estrogen is made mostly in the ovaries, although your adrenal glands make small amounts of this hormone, and so does fat tissue. Estrogen moves through your blood and acts everywhere in your body.

The body can make too little or too much estrogen. Or, you can take in too much estrogen through birth control pills, BPA's, toxins in your food, and personal care products, or estrogen replacement therapy. You might want to keep track of your symptoms by writing them down each day. Bring this symptom journal to your doctor.

Your body makes three main types of estrogen:

Estradiol (E2): The most common type in women of childbearing age.

Estriol (E3): The main estrogen during pregnancy.

Estrone (E1): The only estrogen your body makes after menopause when menstrual periods stop. Too much of this type of estrogen raises the risk of cancer.

Your estrogen levels change throughout the month. They are highest in the middle of your menstrual cycle and lowest during your period. Estrogen levels also drop at menopause.

Symptoms of Estrogen Imbalance

Low Estrogen:

The most common reason for low estrogen in women is menopause or your ovaries were surgically removed. Symptoms of low estrogen include:

- Menstrual periods that are less frequent or that stop
- Hot flashes (suddenly feeling very warm) and/or night sweats
- Trouble sleeping
- Dryness and thinning of the vagina
- Low sexual desire
- Mood swings
- Dry skin

17

Some women get menstrual migraines -a bad headache right before their menstrual period- because of the drop in estrogen. For men, low estrogen can cause excess belly fat and low sexual desire.

High Estrogen:

In women, excess estrogen can lead to these problems, among others:

- Weight gain, mainly in your waist, hips, and thighs
- Menstrual problems, such as light or heavy bleeding
- Worsening of premenstrual syndrome
- Fibrocystic breasts (non-cancerous breast lumps)
- Fibroids (noncancerous tumors) in the uterus
- Fatigue
- Loss of sex drive
- Feeling depressed or anxious

Troubleshooting Estrogen Imbalances

If you scored 3 or higher on section 4 of the self-assessment, you have too much estrogen, or too much estrogen in relation to progesterone, which is also known as estrogen dominance.

Most women in their 40's and 50's are confused about having estrogen dominance because their estrogen levels are dropping. Even women with low estrogen can have estrogen dominance if their progesterone is low in relation. It is all about the ratios and counterbalances when it comes to hormones.

Solutions for Estrogen Dominance

- Support your Gut and Liver. Optimizing your main detox pathways, your gut and your liver are going to help with the breakdown and removal of excess estrogen. The 21-Day Plan in the back of this book is a great place to start, since it is designed to support detoxification

- Avoid Xenoestrogens. These are "fake" estrogens that are found in our environment. These mimic estrogens and contribute to inflammation and weight gain. Plastic water bottles, straws, store receipts, chemicals in cleaning supplies, cosmetics, conventionally raised animal products, soy, dryer sheets, pesticides and tap water.

- Supplement with calcium-D-glucarate to help accelerate estrogen metabolic product removal, DIM, B Vitamins, and adequate protein to help with estrogen metabolism and removal. Adding fermented foods and probiotics can help as well.

- If overweight, lose weight since body fat is an endocrine organ that produces estrogen, typically Estrone, which is the more carcinogenic form.

- Support progesterone to help with balance

Solutions for Too Little Estrogen

Support the adrenal glands by reducing stress and adding an adrenal supplement. The adrenals secrete DHEA, which can convert to estrogen. As ovarian production declines, we must turn to our adrenals (and our gut) to make estrogen.

Add more dietary fat. Estrogen (and our other steroid hormones) are made from fat. If we do not consume enough fat, hormones will decline.

Add Maca to your smoothies or green drinks. Maca is a powerful herb that can stimulate the body to produce more estrogen if levels are low. It also helps to modulate stress.

Consider early menopause and get some testing done.

Progesterone

Progesterone is the peaceful hormone. It is what keeps us sane, calm, and in control.

Progesterone acts on the GABA receptors in the brain to produce a calming effect that helps you sleep. This action is similar to sleeping pills, anxiety medication and alcohol, which all act on those same GABA receptors. Only with progesterone, there is no hangover. GABA is the primary inhibitory neurotransmitter in the brain and protects us from overstimulation. Those women who have disrupted sleep, waking up between 2 am and 4am in the morning or finding that they are more tired when they wake up than when they went to bed are most likely suffering from a progesterone deficiency.

Progesterone is one of the first female hormones to decline. Along with HGH, progesterone can start dipping as early as the mid-twenties, and it can tank fast.

The early symptoms of low progesterone include irregular periods, irritability, anxiety, sleep disturbances and brain fog.

Fertility and menstruation are largely controlled by progesterone.

Progesterone is secreted by the corpus luteum, a temporary endocrine gland that the female body produces after ovulation during the second half of the menstrual cycle.

Progesterone prepares the endometrium for the potential of pregnancy after ovulation. It triggers the lining to thicken to accept a fertilized egg. It also prohibits the muscle contractions in the uterus that would cause the body to reject an egg. While the body is producing high levels of progesterone, the body will not ovulate.

If the woman does not become pregnant, the corpus luteum breaks down, lowering the progesterone levels in the body. This change sparks menstruation. If the body does conceive, progesterone continues to stimulate the body to provide the blood vessels in the endometrium that will feed the growing fetus. The hormone also prepares the lining of the uterus further, so it can accept the fertilized egg.

Once the placenta develops, it also begins to secrete progesterone, supporting the corpus luteum. This causes the levels to remain elevated throughout the pregnancy, so the body does not produce more eggs. It also helps prepare the breasts for milk production.

Women who have low levels of progesterone will have abnormal menstrual cycles or may struggle to conceive because the progesterone does not trigger the proper environment for a conceived egg to grow. Women who have low progesterone levels and who do succeed in getting pregnant are at higher risk for miscarriage or pre-term delivery because the hormone helps maintain the pregnancy.

Stress is often a reason for low progesterone. When we are stressed, our brain gets the message that the danger is near and pumps out cortisol. The innate intelligence of the body knows that times of danger and famine are not the best times to bring a baby into the world, so it may not send the ovaries the message to release an egg. No ovulation means no progesterone production.

Signs of low progesterone include:

- Abnormal uterine bleeding
- Irregular or missed periods
- Spotting and abdominal pain during pregnancy
- Frequent miscarriages
- Premenstrual fluid retention and weight gain
- Anxiety and Panic Attacks
- Cystic Breasts
- Difficulty sleeping
- Brain Fog
- Low Sex Drive
- Saggy, thin skin

In addition, low progesterone levels can cause too-high levels of estrogen (otherwise known as estrogen dominance), which can decrease sex drive, contribute to weight gain, or cause gallbladder problems.

The good news is that progesterone deficiency is easy to fix when you know what to do.

Solutions for Low Progesterone

- Reduce Stress. I know, I sound like a broken record, but stress really messes with your hormones. Practice breathing exercises, gratitude, prayer, read a book, do yoga, go for a leisurely walk.

- Consider Adrenal Support as adrenal health and progesterone go hand in hand.

- Since progesterone stimulates GABA, which calms us, low progesterone can lead to anxiety and insomnia. Using a liposomal GABA supplement can ease the anxiety.

- Supplement with Black Cohosh and Vitex, also green tea extract, DIM and calcium D-glucarate for three months. If help is still needed, consider a bio-identical progesterone cream.

Testosterone

After spending years as an athlete and personal trainer, talk of boosting testosterone was common among my male counterparts. We often equate testosterone with big muscular men, with facial hair, deep voices, and high sex drives.

Testosterone is a hormone generally considered important for men, but did you know it is also a vital hormone for women?

In fact, low T is fairly common in women, especially moms and women over 30. Unfortunately, the symptoms of low testosterone in women are often passed off as just part of getting older, but they shouldn't be.

Many of the women I work with have been to their primary care doctors with symptoms of low testosterone. And their doctors passed off their complaints as a natural part of getting older. Some were sent on their way, while others were handed a prescription for antidepressants.

Hardly a solution!

Here are 6 of the more common symptoms of low testosterone in women:

22

Fatigue

This is one of the top complaints from the moms I work with. Now, if you have a newborn, even if your hormones are in tip-top shape, chances are your sleep is lacking and that is the reason for fatigue.

However, if your kids are older or if you're constantly tired, even when you're able to get a full night's sleep, you could be experiencing one of the symptoms of low testosterone in women. Decreased testosterone levels may contribute to you feeling exhausted and drained.

You may even find it difficult to sleep through the night (even when your kids do). Disrupted sleep is another common symptom for women with low testosterone and/or estrogen and progesterone imbalances. A healthy hormonal balance is key to achieving consistent, restful sleep.

Weight Gain & Difficulty Losing Weight

Many women with low testosterone experience loss of muscle and progressive weight gain.

For women, midlife weight gain is so common that we can often assume it's just part of getting older. I've said this before and I will say it again: Just because something is common does not mean that it's normal. If, out of nowhere, you find yourself unable to control your weight or have changes in muscle tone and bone density, you may be exhibiting symptoms of low testosterone.

Decreased Interest in Sex

Just like in men, testosterone affects sexual arousal in women. Low testosterone can affect women's sex lives in a few different ways. First, there is a general disinterest in sex. As wives, we may find ourselves conflicted because we truly love and are attracted to our husbands, but just have no desire for intimacy. This reduced sex drive, accompanied by dissatisfaction with our own physical appearance can really put a damper on the bedroom activities. And, to make matters worse, another symptom of low testosterone is vaginal dryness, which causes painful intercourse: a not-so-perfect storm in the relationship department.

23

Mood Swings, Depression and Anxiety

If you are experiencing sudden bouts of depression, unexplained mood swings or a generally low mood, then you may be suffering from low testosterone or another hormonal imbalance.

Testosterone plays an important role in mood regulation in the body, and low levels of testosterone can really mess with your mood and confidence. If you are considering taking antidepressants to deal with your depression, then you may want to examine your hormonal health first to see if imbalances in testosterone, estrogen and progesterone are the real cause of your crappy mood.

Low testosterone can be to blame for severe depressive episodes, unpredictable mood swings, or a general "blah" feeling, or simply feeling down. Before letting your primary care doctor write an Rx for an antidepressant, investigate your hormone health and seek a more natural and long-term solution.

In addition to mood swings, low testosterone can trigger anxiety and panic attacks. Mood disturbances occur because testosterone plays a vital role in the regulation of brain chemistry, and a lack of it can trigger mood related symptoms.

Hair Loss

Hair loss is one of the more obvious symptoms of low testosterone. And for women, it can be one of the most devastating. For many women, a bad hair day is simply a bad day!

Although hair loss from low testosterone will be most obvious on the head, hair loss can also occur on other areas of the body.

If you notice that you have to shave your legs and armpits fewer times per month than normal, or if you notice that your hair is getting patchy, you may be suffering from low testosterone. (Okay, so this part about less body hair isn't really a negative. Who enjoys shaving their legs anyway?)

Testosterone is one of the main hormones that support healthy hair production and maintenance. This symptom most often manifests as patchy hair cover on the head or even baldness in women.

Hair loss can also be due to poor nutrition, stress, a traumatic event, pregnancy or a thyroid dysfunction, so it is a good idea to use a holistic approach to balancing hormones like I explain in this book.

Low Bone Density

Testosterone plays a pivotal role in maintaining strong bones. Testosterone deficiency in women often increases the risk of developing osteoporosis, a potentially dangerous condition that can lead to serious bone fractures and loss of independence. And a hip fracture in older women can often lead to a lower life expectancy.

Of course, these are only the most common symptoms, and many of these symptoms can be a result of a combination of dysfunctions in the body.

Solutions for Low Testosterone:

- Intermittent Fasting: What is one of the biggest intermittent fasting benefits? It's been shown to increase testosterone by nearly 200 percent.

- High Intensity Interval Training and Resistance Training: No pink Dumbbells! Lifting heavy weights for 6–12 reps with larger muscle groups like your quadriceps, hamstrings, back, shoulders and chest will help your body pack on the maximum amount of muscle. Specifically, lifting at least 30 minutes up to as long as an hour or so can be very, very beneficial, boosting low testosterone levels. High Intensity Interval Training (HIIT) sessions of as little as 10 minutes are also effective at boosting testosterone levels.

- Eat Healthy Fats: Again, our steroid hormones are made out of cholesterol, so without dietary fat, we will lack some of the raw materials to produce our hormones.

- Liver Detox: Your liver is so crucial to testosterone levels. When your liver does not function optimally, it affects your testosterone output. That's because the liver holds an enzyme that conjugates the 17-beta-hydroxyl group of testosterone. The 21 Days to Hormone Harmony plan at the end of this book will give you a great liver detox.

- Support other hormones
- Balance Blood Sugar
- Evaluate PCOS
- Reduce Stress

CHAPTER 4:

The StressHormone

"Feelings come and go like clouds in a windy sky.
Conscious breathing is my anchor."

—Thích Nh't H'nh

Cortisol - The Stress Hormone

Aside from the big three (estrogen, progesterone and testosterone), cortisol is one of the most popular hormones. Who doesn't remember those late-night commercials that told us that "cortisol causes belly fat". They were right, but that was where the facts ended. Unfortunately, there is no magic pill you can take to regulate cortisol and magically melt belly fat.

Cortisol is often called the "stress hormone" because of its connection to the stress response. However, cortisol is much more than just a hormone released during stress. Understanding cortisol and its effect on the body will help you balance all of your hormones and achieve good health.

Cortisol is one of the steroid hormones and is made in the adrenal glands. Most cells within the body have cortisol receptors. Secretion of the hormone is controlled by the hypothalamus, the pituitary gland, and the adrenal gland, a combination of glands often referred to as the HPA axis.

What does cortisol do?

Because most bodily cells have cortisol receptors, it affects many different functions in the body. Cortisol can help control blood sugar levels, regulate metabolism, help reduce inflammation, and assist with memory formulation. It has a controlling effect on salt and water balance and helps control blood pressure. In women, cortisol also supports the developing fetus during pregnancy. All of these functions make cortisol a crucial hormone to protect overall health and wellbeing.

Cortisol and the Stress Response

Our bodies have a built-in surveillance system for our protection. When the brain perceives a threat, any type of threat, it initiates the stress response via the HPA axis. The word axis refers to a series of signals. So the hypothalamus talks to the pituitary, and then the pituitary sends a message to the adrenal glands telling them to make hormones.

The stress response, which causes a release of cortisol, is initially protective, and it is a good thing. It helps us to deal with and manage our stressors. But this long-term adaptation comes with a price, and that price is decreased health.

You've probably heard "long term stress is bad for your health." But that's pretty vague, right? Thousands of other things are "bad for your health", so how is this different?

Why is stress bad and what symptoms can long term stress cause? To understand this, you need to understand what a normal, healthy stress response is.

This is what's supposed to happen in your body when you get stressed:

When humans became stressed thousands of years ago, it was typically because they were in imminent danger (think of a life or death situation). Maybe a lion was chasing them, or they were starving and had to find food.

In stressful situations like these, the brain only wants to focus on survival and getting out of danger. So the brain signals a normal stress response, which includes telling the adrenal glands to secrete more cortisol, which is also known as the "stress hormone".

The increased cortisol output raises heart rate, increases alertness and makes you stronger, faster and smarter so you can escape danger. It also tells the body to stop focusing on things it doesn't need right now to survive, like digesting food, sleeping, and defending against disease.

Elevated cortisol will also activate the body's own opioid production to dull any pain sensations, making it possible to fight your way out of danger, even if injured.

So in a stressful situation, you get amped up to escape the lion or find food. When the danger has passed, you go back into a relaxed state with normal, healthy cortisol levels. *Cue the music.*

Today, different types of stress mean VERY different outcomes. You might deal with things like excelling in your career, taking care of family, bills and financial burden, relationships, school, deciding what clothes to wear, traffic, staying on schedule, etc. Even WORRYING about something since imagining a future situation in your mind can cause stress and raise cortisol levels.

Do you notice a trend here? These are all everyday things that you take for granted, which keeps you stressed all day long. When you're stressed for longer periods of time, cortisol levels stay elevated.

And it's important to know that your body is designed to be a precisely balanced machine. When cortisol levels increase above normal, this balance is thrown off and there are some major downsides. Such as...

- Trouble sleeping
- Sudden weight gain, regardless of diet and exercises
- Bloating, gas, indigestion
- Low testosterone
- Female hormone imbalances and PMS symptoms
- Brain damage (confusion, forgetfulness, difficulty focusing)
- Getting sick and feeling "under the weather" frequently
- Depression
- Muscle loss

Yikes! Remember, when you're stressed, your body thinks a lion is chasing you. It's only focused on survival and escaping the lion (or other stressors).

So, sleeping, digesting food, burning fat, having sex, and fighting bacteria are all of a sudden not so important for your body. And you're smart enough to know that this isn't ideal in the long-term.

Despite all of this, you may actually still feel pretty good with high cortisol levels. That's because cortisol increases energy, decreases inflammation, and can make you feel awake and alert for very long bouts of time. You can often still juggle whatever life throws at you with high cortisol levels, despite some nagging symptoms.

But cortisol levels can't stay high forever - and that's when REAL problems begin.

But before I tell you why low cortisol levels usually lead to even worse outcomes, I want you to understand why women tend to end up with low cortisol levels.

When you're stressed out for days, weeks, or months, your brain still thinks a lion is chasing you all day, every day. Your brain keeps telling your adrenal glands to pump out more and more cortisol without giving time for rest. Eventually something has to give.

When you fall into this pattern, this is what happens:

Your brain becomes DESENSITIZED to stress.

The brain begins to realize that there is no lion. Much like in the story of the little boy who cried wolf, the brain turns off the normal stress response. This results in an inability to deal with stress, chronic inflammation, and unstable blood sugar, among other problematic issues.

Here is the pattern that I see all of the time: Cortisol levels are normal to begin with, and they increase when you are stressed. If you can break from the stress and relax, they go backwards, back down to normal. If you stay stressed for a long time, cortisol levels remain elevated. Eventually, your body can no longer maintain this, and cortisol levels start to drop below normal levels.

LOW cortisol levels are not conducive to health and happiness.

Here are some of the symptoms of low cortisol:

- Low back pain or joint pain that won't go away
- Feeling tired for no known reason
- Unstable blood sugar (feeling jittery, anxiety)
- Allergies
- Food sensitivities
- GI issues

Low cortisol levels also INCREASE the risk for scary DISEASES. This is so important, but so overlooked!

It's known that cortisol is the body's major anti-inflammatory hormone. And it's also known that almost all diseases are rooted in inflammation or closely tied to it.

This includes:

- Cancer
- Alzheimer's
- Autoimmune disease
- Fibromyalgia
- Skin conditions like eczema
- Heart attacks
- And so much more...

When cortisol levels are low, your body really struggles to handle inflammation. So, if you've got low cortisol, plus your immune system is down from all the stress, it's not hard to imagine why this is a bad sign.

That's why prednisone shots (which are like synthetic cortisol) are so effective in the short term. But these can have devastating side effects and can cause your body to stop producing cortisol on its own.

But there's one bigger problem.

Your doctor may have given you a clean bill of health, even if you are suffering from adrenal dysregulation. The problem is that conventional medicine doesn't have the tools to restore the body's optimal cortisol output. There's no pharmaceutical drug that can do this.

When conventional medicine doctors think about cortisol and the adrenal glands, they are only looking for extreme medical conditions, like Addison's Disease or Cushing's Disease. However, these are extremely rare and most people don't suffer from them.

Most doctors also don't take into consideration that cortisol levels are supposed to change throughout the day. You're supposed to wake up with high levels, and they're supposed to decline throughout the day. That's why it's so important to get your levels tested for an entire day. I'll cover my favorite ways to test cortisol in another chapter.

Solutions for Low Cortisol

- Liver and GI detox, identify hidden stressors, infections and inflammation
- Reduce Stress
- Be gentle on your body. If you usually run, walk. If you usually go to CrossFit, try Tai Chi. In our practice, we have found that when women take their foot off the gas a little and give their bodies a break, all the sudden weight falls with less exercise.
- Limit caffeine and alcohol
- Set a consistent bedtime and wake time
- Supplement with Licorice Root to give you a little extra boost from the little cortisol that you do have

Solutions for High Cortisol

- Balance Blood Sugar (the 21 Day Plan at the back of this book will help you to do that)
- Reduce Stress - this goes without saying

32

- Look for hidden infections in the gut, autoimmunity, and viruses that can raise cortisol
- Evaluate relationships, career, and all life situations that are causing stress
- Learn to say no and have some downtime
- Supplement with B Vitamins, Glutathione, and adaptogenic herbs like ashwaghanda

CHAPTER 5:

Blood Sugar Hormones

The first key to living a longer and healthier life is controlling blood glucose (blood sugar). As I like to joke, it's the 400 lb. gorilla in the room: the obvious truth that is being ignored.

Many well-intentioned folks are constantly seeking the next pill or potion to increase health. But the bottom line is if your blood sugar is out of whack, you'll never maintain significant weight loss or your best health. And since so many Americans suffer from blood sugar challenges, it's an extremely important topic. But why does our blood sugar level have such an impact on overall health? Let me explain.

First, Spikes in blood sugar contribute to accelerated aging.

If you want to age faster than anyone in your neighborhood, simply raise your blood sugar. A repetitive blood sugar roller coaster produces substances called AGEs (Advanced Glycation End Products) via a glycation reaction. AGEs are aptly named since they cause cellular oxidation and inflammation by accelerating the aging process from the inside out, contributing to an array of degenerative diseases. Think of glycation like rust forming on a car bumper, but it's slowly eating away at YOU. Furthermore, constant blood sugar spikes shorten something called telomeres, parts of cells that act as a human "biological clock" and affect how we age. Science has shown that by looking at the length of your telomeres, you can understand the age of your cells. You may be 45 years old, but your telomeres could show your cellular age clocks in at 65. In effect, out of control blood sugar ages you prematurely AND shortens your telomeres, thereby shortening your life.

Second, blood sugar spikes dysregulated hormones.

Hormones are directly affected by our blood sugar levels. And when it comes to anti-aging, weight-loss, and optimal cellular function, hormones are the real answer. Blood sugar spikes equal cellular inflammation, and cellular inflammation equals hormone problems that are typically not solved by taking more hormones.

As an example, think of diabetics: they suffer from cellular membrane inflammation which consequently triggers hormone dysregulation and a host of problems that go with it. To explain, hormone receptors reside on the cell membrane, including receptors to the hormone insulin that allows your body to use glucose for energy. When the cell membrane is inflamed, hormones cannot communicate with the receptor to get the message into the cell where it needs to go for normal function. Simply put, the cell cannot "hear" the message from the hormone insulin to bring the glucose needed for energy into the cell. As a result, glucose builds up in the blood leading to elevated blood sugar levels and more inflammation. This is the state of hormone resistance, or in the case of diabetes, insulin resistance.

Moreover, remember that diabetics do not die of diabetes. Rather, they age prematurely and develop other inflammatory diseases such as heart disease, stroke, obesity, and more. Diabetics literally age faster at the cellular level, evidenced by outward signs such as age spots and wrinkles, and symptoms such as necrosis (lost appendages due to nerve degeneration). Once AGES are produced due to out of control blood sugar, the degeneration process begins, and disease soon follows.

Most diabetics end up with thyroid problems because the thyroid hormone receptors, like most hormone receptors, are also on the cell membrane and are blunted by glucose driven inflammation. This is why many people who take thyroid hormones and the blood work improves, but they don't feel any better. If the message from the thyroid hormone (T3) can't get in the cell, due to inflammation, then the blood levels of hormones can be normal, but your hair keeps thinning, energy dropping, and weight going up (or at least stalling despite what you eat). You must get to the real cause.

Hormones can be crutches but are not a long-term lasting answer. I'd like to emphasize that regenerating and decreasing inflammation of the cell membrane are so important that they are included as two of the five steps in my 5R's of True Cellular Detox and Healing™ approach I use to get very sick clients well.

There are two hormones involved in blood sugar regulation: insulin and glucagon. First, we'll discuss Insulin.

Insulin

Understanding insulin, what insulin does, and how it affects the body, is important to your overall health.

Insulin is secreted by the pancreas and allows the cells in the muscles, fat and liver to absorb glucose that is in the blood. The glucose serves as energy to these cells or it can be converted into fat when needed. Insulin also affects other metabolic processes, such as the breakdown of fat or protein.

When I mention issues with insulin and blood sugar, most people immediately think Diabetes. The most common problem associated with insulin is diabetes. Diabetes occurs when the body either does not secrete enough insulin or when the body no longer uses the insulin it secretes effectively.

Diabetes falls into two categories:

Type 1 Diabetes occurs when the pancreas cannot produce insulin sufficiently to meet its own needs. This commonly occurs in children. While an exact cause has not been found, many consider it to be an autoimmune disease. Some symptoms of Type 1 Diabetes include tiredness, increased urination and thirst, and problems with vision.

Type 2 Diabetes is more commonly associated with adults and lifestyle choices. People with Type 2 Diabetes will produce insulin, but often not enough for their body's needs. They may also struggle to use the insulin they produce effectively. People usually don't even know they have Type 2 Diabetes until they have an annual checkup, as symptoms tend to be mild until the disease has become severe.

When the body does not produce enough insulin or use it efficiently, blood sugar levels build in the body. When this happens, the body's cells do not receive the energy they need from glucose, so you may struggle with fatigue. Blood sugar may be confusing sometimes, because we look at food and it can be hard to determine which is good and which is not.

Imagine you go into the break room at work. You see a bowl of fruit and a tray of donuts. We see sugar in both the donut and apple. They both have sugar and they're both sweet. But we know that the apple is actually much better for us because it contains some other nutrients that the body can use - like vitamins and minerals and fiber. The fiber is actually what really protects the body from that insulin and glucose spike. (Unless the apple has been genetically modified to contain more sugar and less fiber. But that's a whole other story, perhaps for another book.)

What I'm talking about is that understanding how your hormones in your body help keep blood sugar in balance can really save your life. That knowledge is really powerful because even while blood sugar imbalances are so common, they can lead to serious disease imbalances, and chronic conditions.

Having good blood sugar balance is, I have to say, one of the most important benchmarks of overall wellness because it prevents other kinds of imbalances from happening that can actually threaten your life. Thyroid health, adrenal health, Growth Hormone, Estrogen, and Cortisol are just a few of the hormones that you can be affected by poor blood sugar balance.

Now we'll discuss glucagon - Insulin's Perfect Match

Your hormones do a fabulous job of keeping the blood sugar in balance though a natural process called homeostasis.

Here is how it works:

Our blood sugar goes up after we eat.

Insulin is released to bring it back down to our normal range.

So normally, if you haven't eaten recently, your blood sugar should be between 70 and 120.

We actually have some backup stores of blood sugar in case we haven't eaten in a longer period of time. So if we eat a carbohydrate filled meal, some of that sugar will be broken into glucose and the rest of it will actually be stored in the liver as glycogen.

When the time comes that the brain senses that your blood sugar is getting low, it calls on the pancreas again. This time it's not asking for a release of insulin, it's actually triggering the release of glucagon. When glucagon is released, its job is to tell the liver to release its stored glycogen. Glycogen then gets broken down into glucose, your blood sugar rises and so there you have it – balance.

There's also another equally fabulous backup system for when you run out of glycogen and you run out of glucose. It's your fat!

Fat is stored energy. In the absence of glucose and glycogen stores, you'll actually start breaking your fat into fatty acids and ketone bodies. Glucose, fatty acids, and ketone bodies are going to be made from your fat through your body's amazing process called ketosis.

If you have a healthy, well-functioning system, you will always keep your blood sugar in balance, whether you're fasting, whether you're on a Keto Diet or whether you're eating a well-balanced meal. Hopefully, that helps you understand how ketosis works, how insulin works, and how glucagon works. Basically, just know your body is going to do everything it can to keep balance.

The following are just some basic foundations when it comes to lifestyle practices to help balance your blood sugar and insulin.

Diet and Lifestyle Tools for Managing Blood Sugar

- **Keep Simple Carbs Low**. You don't have to go "no carb" or even low carb, just choose complex carbs like an apple, sweet potato or vegetables rather than a donut. Keeping carbs below 100 grams per day is a good number to shoot for. Start with the diet in the back of this book to help balance blood sugar (and the rest of your hormones at the same time).

- **Exercise Daily**. High Intensity Interval Training will make your cells more sensitive to insulin and 10-minute walks before or after meals can really help to keep blood sugar stable.*

- **Eat Moderate (Not High) Protein**. Most people do not realize that protein, consumed in excess, will get converted to sugar through a process called gluconeogenesis.

- **Fast**. Going longer periods of time without food can train your body to become more sensitive to insulin.

- **Stress Reduction**. Stress raises cortisol and cortisol raises blood sugar. Practice deep breathing and focus on breathing from your belly, rather than your chest. This one simple shift can reduce the body's perception of stress significantly enough to lower blood sugar. Additionally, try practicing daily stress reducing rituals such as meditation, yoga, Qi Gong, reading, playing sports, art or connecting with friends.

- **Supplementation**. The following supplements are proven safe and effective for improving blood sugar balance and insulin sensitivity:
  a. Omega 3 Fatty Acids
  b. Berberine and Cinnamon
  c. Garlic - Adiponectin Modulator
  d. Magnesium and Chromium

*A note regarding exercise for blood sugar control:

Exercise helps reduce inflammation and blood glucose. So when you exercise, it causes your cells to become more sensitive to insulin. Exercise also reduces stress, which helps prevent inflammation and the production of stress hormones (like cortisol) that also raise your blood sugar level.

Just 15 minutes of exercise can decrease your blood glucose levels. If your blood sugar is getting high when you eat, go exercise. Going for a walk after dinner will really help to stabilize your blood sugar. Your goal should be at least 30 minutes of exercise, five days a week. And if you exercise before or after a meal, it promotes better insulin sensitivity and you're actually able to further stabilize your blood sugar.

CHAPTER 6:

Thyroid Hormones

Y our thyroid, one of the largest endocrine glands, greatly influences almost every cell in your body. Aside from regulating your metabolism
and weight by controlling the fat-burning process, thyroid hormones are
also required for the growth and development in children, brain and neuro-
logical development in babies and in nearly every physiological process in
your body.

When your thyroid levels are out of balance, so are you. Too much or
too little hormone secretion in this gland can spell trouble for your overall
health and wellbeing.

Poor thyroid function has been linked to serious health conditions like
fibromyalgia, irritable bowel syndrome, acne, eczema, gum disease, infertility, and autoimmune diseases, which is why it's imperative that you learn
how your thyroid works and what can cause it to go off kilter.

The Thyroid Gland: Understanding How It Works

The thyroid gland is a butterfly-shaped gland found inside your neck,
right under your larynx or voice box. A two-inch long, brownish red, highly vascular gland, it has two lobes located on each side of the windpipe that
are both connected by a tissue called the isthmus. A normal thyroid gland
weighs somewhere between 20 and 60 grams. Your thyroid is responsible for
producing the master metabolism hormones that control every function in
your body. It produces three types of hormones:

- Triiodothyronine (T3)

- Thyroxine (T4)

- Diiodothyronine (T2)

40

Hormones secreted by your thyroid interact with all your other hormones, including insulin, cortisol, and sex hormones like estrogen, progesterone, and testosterone. The fact that these hormones are all tied together and are in constant communication explains why a less-than-optimal thyroid status is associated with so many widespread symptoms and diseases.

Almost 90 percent of the hormone produced by your thyroid is in the form of T4, the inactive form. Your liver then converts the T4 into T3, the active form, with the help of an enzyme. We don't currently know much about T2, and it is the subject of a number of ongoing studies, but I want you to know it exists. But that is all I will say about it for now.

If everything is working properly, you will make what you need and have the correct amounts of T3 and T4, which control the metabolism of every cell in your body. If your T3 is inadequate, either by scarce production or not converting properly from T4, your whole system suffers. T3 is critically important because it tells the nucleus of your cells to send messages to your DNA to rev up your metabolism by burning fat. This is how T3 lowers cholesterol levels, regrows hair, and helps keep you lean.

Your T3 levels can be disrupted by nutritional imbalances, toxins, allergens, infections, and stress, and this can lead to a series of complications, including thyroid cancer, hypothyroidism and hyperthyroidism, which today are three of the most prevalent thyroid-related diseases.

Now, let's discuss and delve deeper into these thyroid problems.

Hypothyroidism: Sluggish Thyroid Syndrome

Hypothyroidism occurs when your thyroid produces too little thyroid hormone, a condition often linked to iodine deficiency. In addition, 10 percent of the general population in the United States, and 20 percent of women over age 60, have "subclinical" hypothyroidism, meaning your symptoms aren't bad enough to treat, and only slightly abnormal according to lab tests.

Unfortunately, only a small percentage of these women are being treated. The reason behind this is the misinterpretation and misunderstanding of lab tests, particularly TSH (thyroid stimulating hormone). Most physicians believe that if your TSH value is within the "normal" range, your thyroid is fine. But as my dad always said, "the devil is in the details". More and more physicians (the good ones, at least) are now discovering that the TSH value is truly unreliable for diagnosing hypothyroidism, and that it is not measuring thyroid function at all.

How to Know If You Are Hypothyroid

Identifying hypothyroidism and its cause can be tricky. Many of the symptoms of hypothyroidism are vague and overlap with other hormonal imbalances and disorders. As well, physicians often miss a thyroid problem since they rely on just a few traditional tests, leaving other clues undetected. And new moms and perimenopausal women are among the populations where hypothyroidism is most often missed. Unfortunately, doctors can too easily blame "busy lifestyles", "demanding jobs" and "babies who don't yet sleep through the night" for most of the symptoms these struggling women come to them with.

People with a sluggish thyroid usually experience:

Lethargy. Fatigue and lack of energy are typical signs of thyroid dysfunction. Depression has also been linked to the condition. If you've been diagnosed with depression, make it a point that your physician checks your thyroid levels.

It's essential to note that not all tiredness or lack of energy can be blamed on a dysfunctional thyroid gland.

Thyroid-related fatigue begins to appear when you cannot sustain energy long enough, especially when compared to a past level of fitness or ability. If your thyroid foundation is weak, sustaining energy output is going to be a challenge. You will notice you just don't seem to have the energy to do the things like you used to.

Some of the obvious signs of thyroid fatigue include:

• Feeling like you don't have the energy to exercise, and typically not exercising on a consistent basis

- A heavy or tired head, especially in the afternoon; your head is a very sensitive indicator of thyroid hormone status

- Falling asleep as soon as you sit down when you don't have anything to do

- Weight gain – Easy weight gain or difficulty losing weight, despite an aggressive exercise program and watchful eating, is another indicator

- Rough and scaly skin and/or dry, coarse, and tangled hair. If you have perpetually dry skin that doesn't respond well to moisturizing lotions or creams, consider hypothyroidism as a factor.

- Hair loss. Women should especially pay close attention to their thyroid when unexplained hair loss occurs. Fortunately, if your hair loss is due to low thyroid function, your hair will come back quickly with proper thyroid treatment.

- Sensitivity to cold. Feeling cold all the time is also a sign of low thyroid function. Hypothyroid people are slow to warm up, even in a sauna, and don't sweat with mild exercise.

- Low basal temperature. Another telltale sign of hypothyroidism is a low basal body temperature (BBT), less than 97.6 ° F (36.4° C) averaged over a minimum of three days. It is best to get a BBT thermometer to assess this and take your temperature first thing in the morning before you get out of bed.

Any of these symptoms can be suggestive of an underactive thyroid. The more of these symptoms you have, the higher the likelihood you have hypothyroidism. Furthermore, if you have someone in your family with any of the following conditions, your risk of a thyroid problem becomes higher:

- Goiter

- Diabetes

- Multiple sclerosis (MS)

- Prematurely gray hair
- Autoimmune diseases, (i.e. rheumatoid arthritis, lupus, sarcoidosis, Sjogren's)
- Elevated cholesterol levels
- Left-handedness
- Crohn's disease or ulcerative colitis
- High or low thyroid function

The more vigilant you are in assessing your own symptoms and risk factors, and then presenting the complete picture to your physician, the easier it will be for you to get the proper treatment.

What about Overactive Thyroid?

Thyroxine or T4 is a hormone made by the thyroid gland carried throughout your body in your bloodstream. Many of your cells and tissues depend on thyroxine to work properly.

An overactive thyroid secretes too much T4, causing some of your body functions to accelerate. Physicians may use the term "thyrotoxicosis" instead of "hyperthyroidism." This condition is more common in women; about eight in 100 women and one 1 in 100 men develop hyperthyroidism at some point in their lives, and it can occur at any age.

Symptoms of hyperthyroidism:

- Feeling restless, nervous, emotional, and irritable
- Sleeping poorly, and feel as if you're always on the go
- Difficulty concentrating
- Frequent bowel movements
- Irregular menstrual periods in women
- Weight loss (or weight gain, in rare cases)
- Rapid, forceful, or irregular heartbeat
- Lack of menstrual periods in women
- Protruding eyes or exophthalmos

Some of these symptoms may be unnoticeable at first and then become worse as your thyroxine levels start to shoot up higher.

Untreated hyperthyroidism can lead to heart problems like atrial fibrillation, cardiomyopathy, angina, and heart failure. Hyperthyroid women can potentially have difficulty giving birth.

Diagnosing a Thyroid Issue

There are a few ways to diagnose an underactive or hyperactive thyroid. I prefer using the following laboratory tests if you want to get the real score of your thyroid health:

Thyroid Labs: The Functional Medicine Version

A functional medicine look at your thyroid is more in depth than just a TSH and maybe a T4. We do a broader range of tests and look at a narrower range of optimal results. Here are some of the labs I run on my patients, what they actually mean, and what kind of results are ideal:

TSH

Thyroid-stimulating hormone is released from your pituitary gland to communicate with your thyroid. If your TSH is high, it's sort of like your brain shouting at your thyroid to work harder. Research has linked a lab "normal" TSH of 2.5-3.5 U/mL with a 69% risk of dying from a heart attack or stroke. Now you can see why the optimal (functional) range is so important for your health.

Lab range: .45-5.5 U/mL

Optimal range: 0.6 -1.9 U/mL

Total T4

T4 is mostly metabolically inactive in the body and has to be converted to T3 to be usable. This lab gives you a total of unbound and bound forms of T4. Hormones have to be unbound from the protein carrier to be used by your body. Because of this, this lab doesn't give us the activity of T4 when measured alone. T4 is measured in conjunction with a T3 uptake.

Reference Range: 4.5-12 mcg/DL

Optimal range: 6.0-12.0 mcg/DL

T3 Uptake

This lab doesn't look directly at T3, but is very useful at indirectly looking at other hormones such as estrogen or testosterone and their relation with the binding of thyroid hormones.

Reference range: 22-35%

Optimal range: 28-38%

Total T3

This lab shows us the total amount of metabolically active thyroid hormone. It allows a doctor to check your body's ability to convert T4 to T3 and to rule out an overactive thyroid.

Reference Range: 80-200 ng/DL

Optimal range: 100-180 ng/DL

Free T4

This will tell you the levels of free or active form of T4. This will be low in cases of hypothyroidism but can be normal in subclinical, early stages of thyroid dysfunction.

Reference Range: 0.8-1.8 ng/DL

Optimal range: 1.09-1.9 ng/DL

Free T3

This is the more active, usable form of your thyroid hormone. Low T3 syndromes are a common dysfunction that I see in my practice and a low level of this hormone is strongly linked to a higher risk of a heart attack. The problem is that if you're taking a synthetic T4 medication, your body isn't converting the hormone properly into T3. However, there are many reasons your thyroid medication may not be working.

Reference Range: 2.3-4.2 pg/mL

Optimal range: 2.3-4.5 pg/mL

Reverse T3

Chronic stress and high cortisol can raise levels of reverse T3, which is an unusable form of the thyroid hormone.

Reference Range: 90-350 pg/ml

Optimal range: 100-320 pg/ml

Thyroid Antibodies

High levels of thyroid antibodies show an autoimmune attack against the thyroid. The overwhelming majority of low thyroid cases are on the autoimmune spectrum, the most common being Hashimoto's disease.

Thyroid Peroxidase (TPO) Ab optimal range: 0-0 IU/mL

Thyroglobulin Ab optimal range: 0-0.9 IU/mL

In addition to these thyroid-focused labs, functional medicine practitioners are likely to recommend additional labs to address your microbiome, immune system, and other hormones. These should also be considered for the most complete picture of what is going on with your health.

Getting the big picture from lab work is a solid first step towards finding out exactly what is going on with your thyroid. What conventional doctors may not tell you is that there are many thyroid dysfunctions that typically don't show up on labs, and that throwing synthetic thyroid medication at the problem will, in many cases, not do enough to relieve symptoms. Luckily, you can do more to help.

Basal Body Temperature

Although there are a few different protocols, the most commonly used is a measure of your basal body temperature at rest first thing in the morning over three days to determine average basal body temperature.

TRH Stimulation Test

For more difficult cases, TRH can be measured using the TRH stimulation test. TRH helps identify hypothyroidism that's caused by inadequacy of the pituitary gland.

Other tests that might be indicated for more complex cases are a thyroid scan, fine-needle aspiration and thyroid ultrasound. But these are specialized tests that your physician will use only in a small number of cases or in special situations.

Even if all your lab tests turn out normal, you still likely have subclinical hypothyroidism if you have multiple thyroid symptoms.

What About Thyroid Cancer?

According to the National Cancer Institute at the National Institutes of Health, there are an estimated 60,220 new cases and 1,850 deaths from thyroid cancer in the United States alone. Thyroid cancer is classified into four different types: papillary thyroid cancer, follicular thyroid cancer, medullary thyroid cancer and anaplastic thyroid cancer.

As with any type of cancer, early intervention heightens your chances of remission and recovery. This is why you should always be on the lookout for clues. Below is a list of potential warning signs of thyroid cancer from Roswell Park Cancer Institute:

- Unusual lumps, nodules, bumps or swelling in the neck
- Pain in the front of the neck or throat
- Hoarseness or other voice changes that do not go away
- A constant cough that is not due to a cold

The Cancer Treatment Centers of America explains that there are certain components that may heighten an individual's overall risk for this disease. These include:

Gender

Females are three times more vulnerable to developing thyroid cancer than males. Papillary thyroid cancer is typically found in women of childbearing age.

Age

Two-thirds of thyroid cancer cases occur between ages 20 and 55.

Family History

Familial medullary thyroid cancer, which is a rare type of thyroid cancer, is caused by an inherited mutation in the RET proto-oncogene. If you have inherited this gene mutation from your parents, your likelihood of contracting this disease is twice as high as other people.

As well, having someone in the family with goiter, thyroid cancer or other thyroid-related diseases increases one's risk.

Iodine Deficiency

Iodine is an essential ingredient for the secretion of thyroid hormones. A deficiency in this nutrient can impair the thyroid significantly.

Environment

Individuals who are exposed excessively or repeatedly to radiation, including routine diagnostic X-rays (i.e. chest or dental X-ray) and other radioactive materials are, especially during childhood, more likely to incur thyroid cancer and/or other forms of cancer.

4 Things that Wreck your Thyroid

These are some key contributing factors that can ruin your healthy thyroid function:

Gluten. Gluten, along with other food sensitivities, is a notorious culprit of thyroid dysfunction as they cause inflammation. Gluten causes autoimmune responses in many people and can be responsible for Hashimoto's thyroiditis, a common autoimmune thyroid condition. Approximately 30 percent of the people with Hashimoto's thyroiditis have an autoimmune reaction to gluten and it usually goes unrecognized.

A gluten sensitivity can cause your gastrointestinal system to malfunction. So foods you eat aren't completely digested, often leading to leaky gut syndrome. These food particles can then be absorbed into your blood-stream, where your body misidentifies them as antigens – substances that shouldn't be there – and then produces antibodies against them.

These antigens look similar to the molecules in your thyroid gland. In a case of mistaken identity, your body accidentally attacks your thyroid. This is known as an autoimmune reaction in which your body actually attacks itself.

Testing can be done for gluten and other food sensitivities, which involves measuring your IgG and IgA antibodies.

I prefer an elimination diet where gluten is removed for several months and we measure improvement in thyroid symptoms and lab markets. If symptoms improve during the elimination period and return when gluten is reintroduced, a diagnosis of non-celiac gluten sensitivity (NCGS) can be made.

Soy. Believe it or not, soy is not the wholesome health food the agricultural and food companies have led you to believe.

When my son Paxton was in the NICU as a newborn, I had to fight a team of doctors and nurses to prevent Paxton and the other preemies from being force-fed this neurotoxic, endocrine disrupting substance.

Virtually thousands of scientific studies now link soy foods to malnutrition, digestive stress, immune system weakness, cognitive decline, reproductive disorders, infertility, and a host of other problems, on top of the damage it causes your thyroid. Soy phytoestrogens are potent anti-thyroid agents that cause hypothyroidism and may cause thyroid cancer. In infants, consumption of soy formula has been linked to autoimmune thyroid disease.

Don't worry my vegan sisters. Properly fermented, organic, and unprocessed soy products such as natto, miso, and tempeh are fine to consume; it's the unfermented soy products that you should stay away from, like soy meat, soy milk, soy cheese, etc.

Bromines. Bromines are a common endocrine disruptor. Because bromide is also a halide, it competes for the same receptors that are used in the thyroid gland to capture iodine. This will inhibit thyroid hormone production resulting in a low thyroid state.

When you ingest or absorb bromine, it displaces iodine, and this iodine deficiency leads to an increased risk for cancer of the breast, thyroid gland, ovary, and prostate – cancers that we see at alarmingly high rates today.

In addition to psychiatric and thyroid problems, bromine toxicity can manifest as skin rashes and severe acne, loss of appetite and abdominal pain, fatigue, a metallic taste in your mouth, and cardiac arrhythmias.

Bromine can be found regularly in a number of places, including:

- Pesticides, specifically methyl bromide, used mainly on strawberries, predominantly in California
- Plastics, such as those used to make computers
- Bakery goods and some flours often contain a "dough conditioner" called potassium bromate
- Soft drinks, including Mountain Dew, Gatorade, Sun Drop, Squirt, Fresca, and other citrus-flavored sodas, in the form of brominated vegetable oils (BVOs)
- Fire retardants like polybromo diphenyl ethers or PBDEs is used in fabrics, carpets, upholstery, and mattresses

The more you can free your body of this toxin, the more iodine your body will be able to hang onto, and the better your thyroid will function.

You can help your body detox from bromine and fluoride exposure by doing the following:

- Increase your iodine and vitamin C intake
- Opt for unrefined sea salt
- Have Epsom salts baths
- Sweat in a far-infrared sauna

Stress and Adrenal Function. Stress is one of the worst thyroid offenders. Your thyroid function is intimately tied to your adrenal function, which is intimately affected by how you handle stress.

Most of us are almost always under chronic stress, which results in increased adrenaline and cortisol levels. Elevated cortisol has a negative impact on thyroid function. Thyroid hormone levels drop during stressful times when you actually need it the most.

When stress becomes chronic, the flood of stress chemicals – adrenaline and cortisol – produced by your adrenal glands interfere with your thyroid hormones, causing a whole gamut of health-related issues like obesity, high blood pressure, high cholesterol, and/or unstable blood sugar levels. A prolonged stress response can lead to adrenal exhaustion, which is also known as adrenal fatigue, which is often found alongside thyroid disease.

But that's not all. Environmental toxins place extra stress on your body too. Pollutants such as petrochemicals, organochlorines, pesticides and chemical food additives negatively affect thyroid function.

5. **Iodine** (The Goldilocks Secret). Iodine could be the biggest piece of the puzzle when it comes to thyroid hormones. It is a vitally important nutrient that is detected in every organ and tissue. It is essential for healthy thyroid function and efficient metabolism, and there is increasing evidence that links it to numerous diseases, including cancer.

Iodine is a potent anti-bacterial, anti-parasitic, anti-viral and anti-cancer agent. It has four significant roles in your body, namely to maintain your weight and metabolism, to develop brain and cognitive function in children, to optimize fertility, and to strengthen your immune system.

Though thyroid health is often what people think of when they think of iodine, other tissues also absorb and use large amounts of iodine, including your breasts, skin, salivary glands, pancreas, brain, stomach, cerebral spinal fluid and thymus.

Iodine deficiency or insufficiency in any of these tissues will lead to tissue dysfunction. Hence, the following symptoms could provide clues that you're not getting enough iodine in your diet:

Salivary glands: Disables your saliva production, making your mouth dry.

Skin: Results in rough and dry skin and inability to sweat normally.

Brain: Lowers alertness and intelligence quotient (IQ) levels.

Muscles: Produces nodules, scar tissue, pain, fibrosis, fibromyalgia.

The Total Diet Study, performed by the FDA, reported an iodine intake reduction from 621 micrograms for two-year-olds between 1974 and 1982, compared with 373 micrograms between 1982 and 1991. During the same time period, the baking industry replaced iodine-based anti-caking agents with bromine-based agents.

In addition to iodine's disappearance from our food supply, exposure to toxic competing halogens – bromine, fluorine, chlorine, and perchlorate – has dramatically increased. You absorb these halogens through your food, water, medications, and environment, and they selectively occupy your iodine receptors, worsening your iodine deficit.

Here are more factors contributing to falling iodine levels:

- Diets low in fish, shellfish and seaweed
- Vegan and vegetarian diets
- Less use of iodide in the food and agricultural industry
- Fluoridated drinking water
- Rocket fuel (perchlorate) contamination in food
- Decreased use of iodized salt
- Less use of iodide in the food and agricultural industry
- Use of radioactive iodine in many medical procedures, which competes with natural iodine

Here are some helpful strategies to increase your iodine levels naturally:

- Eat organic as often as possible. Wash all produce thoroughly to minimize your pesticide exposure.

- Avoid eating or drinking from (or storing food and water in) plastic containers. Use glass and safe ceramic vessels.

- If you have to eat grain, look for organic whole-grain breads and flour. Grind your own grain, if possible. Look for the "no bromine" or "bromine-free" label on commercial baked goods.

- Avoid sodas. Make natural, filtered water your beverage of choice.

- Look for personal care products that aren't laced with toxic chemicals. Remember: anything you put on your skin can potentially go into your bloodstream.

More is not better

If is important to note that with iodine, more is not better. In fact, iodine in large quantities can be used as a treatment to slow or shut down an overactive thyroid, so too much can cause bigger problems.

Let me put that in a different way. The same iodine that you are using in small amounts to boost your thyroid is also used in larger quantities to shut down your thyroid. So be conservative with your dosing and always supplement in combination with selenium for extra protection. To avoid any issues, start with selenium supplementation, 200 mcg per day. Then add iodine at 150-200 mcg per day.

Simple Steps That You Can Do to Improve Your Thyroid Health

- Identify and treat the underlying causes. Find out what's really triggering your thyroid problems – whether it's iodine deficiency, hormone imbalance, environmental toxicity or inflammation – and address it appropriately.

- Load up on fresh iodine-rich foods. As an alternative to iodine supplementation, eat enormous amounts of toxin-free sea vegetables or seaweeds like spirulina, hijiki, wakame, arame, dulse, nori,

54

and kombu, which are loaded with the thyroid-friendly nutrient, iodine, and other beneficial minerals. These can be found in specialty Asian food markets.

- Pay attention to other key aspects of your diet. Munch on Brazil nuts, which are rich in selenium. Load up on foods high in vitamin A and omega-3 fatty acids. Veer away from gluten and soy-containing foods and beverages.

- Minimize your stress levels. Take a break, meditate, soak in the tub, go on vacation – do whatever works for you. Practice Emotional Freedom Technique (EFT), an energy psychology tool that reduces stress extremely well.

- Try to limit your exposure to toxins. Filter your air and water to avoid contact with poisonous contaminants.

- Use an infrared sauna and hot soaks to help your body combat infections and detoxify from petrochemicals, metals, PCBs, pesticides, and mercury. Taking chlorella for detoxification is also advised.

- Avoid all sources of bromide as much as possible - Bromides are a menace to your endocrine system and are present all around you. Despite a ban on the use of potassium bromate in flour by the World Health Organization (WHO), bromides can still be found in some over-the-counter medications, foods, and personal care products. Being a savvy reader of labels can save you from tons of toxic trouble.

- Get adequate amounts of sleep. Inadequate sleep contributes to stress and prevents your body from regenerating fully.

- Exercise. Exercise directly stimulates your thyroid gland to secrete more thyroid hormone and increases the sensitivity of all your tissues to your thyroid hormone. It is even thought that many of the health benefits of exercise stem directly from improved thyroid function.

CHAPTER 7:

The Youth Hormone

We've talked about the sex hormones (estrogen, progesterone and testosterone), the stress hormone (cortisol), and the metabolic hormones (thyroid, insulin, and glucagon).

But the one hormone that tends to get ignored is the Youth Hormone, also known as the Human Growth Hormone or HGH.

What?! I know. How come no one told you about the youth hormone? Don't worry, Girl. I got your back.

As women age, we often think about dropping estrogen levels, tired adrenals and lackluster thyroid function as the major contributing factors to the undesirable signs of aging

However, many of those not-so-sexy traits that we associate with growing old are actually in part a result of dropping HGH levels. If there were ever a hormone you'd want for a best friend, this would be it.

HGH is your BFF!

But wait! I know what you are thinking. Growth Hormone? I don't want to GROW. In fact, I was hoping to do some shrinking (especially around the waist-line).

I get it. That misconception about HGH is fueled by the bodybuilding community who often misuse human growth hormone along with steroids and other anabolic compounds. That isn't at all what we are talking about here.

Human growth hormone (HGH) is actually so much more than a tool to increase muscle mass. In fact, once you learn **all the benefits of**

HGH, you'll probably want to do whatever you can to take advantage of it – legally and naturally, of course.

Let's talk benefits! Optimal HGH levels play a role in:
- Reversing the signs of aging
- Increasing lean muscle mass
- Improving sleep
- Improving mood
- Repairing damaged tissues
- Promoting healthy growth of hair, skin and nails
- Reducing wrinkles and saggy skin
- Decreasing fat tissue
- Increasing bone density
- Heightening Libido
- Increasing fat and sugar metabolism
- Reducing brain fog and improving memory

HGH's effects are so potent it is often referred to as the "Youth Hormone" due to its ability to turn back the clock.

What is Human Growth Hormone?

So what exactly is HGH and what makes it so powerful?

Secreted by the pituitary gland, HGH is an anabolic hormone responsible for spurring growth throughout childhood and adolescence. In other words, it's what makes little babies grow into young adults. It's also the reason why it's so easy to stay lean during those youthful years *(Remember how much we used to be able to eat!)*.

It's responsible for collagen and muscle tissue synthesis, which is one of the major reasons HGH is known for its anti-aging effects, especially with skin texture and elasticity. Loss of HGH is a primary reason why we develop wrinkles, sagging skin and lose hair as we age.

Human Growth Hormone has a potent effect on mood disorders, especially mood swings accompanying unreasonable anger, irritability, anxiety and depression.

Optimizing HGH is especially important for perimenopausal and post-menopausal women as they suffer from increased body fat, decreased muscle tone, sagging skin, brain fog, low libido, depression and joint pain - all of which can be combated by balancing your youth hormone. Optimized HGH levels also help to diminish hot flashes and night sweats.

How to Optimize Your HGH

You are wondering, "How do I know if I need more HGH and how do I prevent my body from losing this precious hormone?"

Well, there are TWO important things to understand:

1. Our natural HGH production begins to decline once we reach our 20s, resulting in a progressive loss of muscle mass and increase in fat tissue.

This loss continues at about 10 to 15 percent each year after the age of 30 and leads to the standard symptoms of aging like sagging skin, loss of energy and endurance, difficulty recovering from injuries, and graying hair (AKA "getting old").

If you are 35 or over and are suffering from any of the symptoms mentioned above, your HGH could use a boost.

2. While HGH injections are an option for the elderly and children with true clinical deficiencies and growth disorders, supplemental injections for health optimization and anti-aging are not readily available and are expensive. You can expect to fork over $2,000 or more per month to get HGH at anti-aging clinics in New York or LA.

There is another population that is using HGH injections: body-builders are buying HGH on the black market and self-injecting. They are often taking too high a dose and stacking their HGH with Steroids or other performance enhancing drugs, and they are often faced with bothersome side effects due to using the hormone improperly. Additionally, obtaining hormones from oversea pharmacies can be risky and even life threatening.

There are many supplements, creams, and even prescription medications that contain precursors to HGH, meaning nutrients or amino acids to help activate the HGH you already have. And none of them have really been proven effective.

Three Human Growth Hormone Stimulators

Luckily, there are several simple ways to naturally boost your levels of HGH without supplements or injections.

HGH Booster #1: Deep Sleep

Human growth hormone is released not in a continuous flow, but in pulses. And some of these major "pulses" occur during deep sleep.

This occurs because growth hormone plays a role in repairing and restoring the body, which often takes place during our slumber. But not just any slumber. Specifically, our brains secrete growth hormone during the third stage of our sleep cycle, when our brain temperature, breathing and heart rates, and blood pressure are all at their lowest levels.

To get to this stage, we have to bypass stage two, which is where most adults usually spend 45 to 50 percent of their time asleep.

To optimize HGH levels, we want to get into that third stage of sleep, also known as the "slow wave" stage. This requires a deep level of sleep that is often interrupted either by our sleep environment, stress, diet, or any one of a number of factors. So to get the growth hormone release we want, we have to employ tactics to help us sleep more deeply, more often.

How to Sleep More Deeply (3 Ways)

Even though we might know that deep sleep is good for us and helps to stimulate growth hormone, getting enough of it can be a real challenge.

Check out these tips for longer, deeper sleep.

1. Soak up the Sun

Sunlight plays a key role in the secretion of melatonin – a hormone produced in the pineal gland responsible for our sleep-wake cycles.

Getting more sunlight during the day naturally helps the body signal the release of melatonin when it gets dark at night. This release makes us feel sleepy and ready for bed.

2. Power down

The seemingly harmless devices we often carry into bed (tablets, phones, etc.) actually work against us when it comes to sleep. The artificial blue light emitted from the screens actually disturbs normal hormone levels, disrupting our sleep cycles. That's why I recommend removing the TV from your bedroom, and also avoiding bright screens 2 to 3 hours before bedtime.

3. Limit caffeine

Obviously, you don't want to guzzle down a fully caffeinated cup of coffee before going to bed, but you should also try to limit caffeine throughout the day. Caffeine messes with your natural hormonal rhythm and metabolism and that can play a role in disrupting sleep.

A few other tricks to getting a deeper sleep include: developing a regular bedtime, supplementing with magnesium, and creating a sleep journal noting anything that affects your sleep.

**This is a little bit like the chicken and the egg, but optimized HGH levels promote better sleep and better sleep promotes more HGH production.

HGH Booster #2: Fasting

Believe it or not, abstaining from eating is also one of the best ways to stimulate human growth hormone. In fact, in one study, fasting caused participants serum growth hormone levels to increase by a whopping 500%!

Don't worry. I'm not talking about embarking on a month-long fast in order to boost growth hormone.

By "fasting", I'm actually referring to what is termed as *intermittent fasting*. This type of fasting involves eating daily, but only in a certain window of time.

For instance, the most popular form of intermittent fasting involves simply skipping breakfast and eating your first meal at lunchtime. In doing this, you'll be performing a daily 14 to 16-hour fast from dinner the night before to lunch the next day.

Okay, let me address the "elephant in the room" here. Many of you have been led to believe that skipping meals slows your metabolism, and that it's best to eat lots of small meals to keep your metabolic fire burning. For many years, I believed this to be true as well, until I started digging into the research.

Let's talk about this.

Studies show that fasting for short periods of time actually has no effect on metabolism. In fact, researchers have found *there is no difference in calories burned over a 24-hour period between people who eat breakfast and those that skip it altogether (Yeah, that trainer at the gym is wrong!)*

The breakfast skipper's metabolism is unharmed by daily fasting and there was no "boosting" of the breakfast eater's metabolisms.

So much for those promises of breakfast "kickstarting" our metabolisms, right?

To try out fasting for yourself, simply start by skipping breakfast a few days a week to see how you feel. One thing to remember, however, is to not ingest any calories during the "fasting" period – no milk or sugar in your tea, no juices, etc.

How to Fast

If your last meal was at 6 p.m., then your fast will begin at 9 p.m. (our bodies take about 3 hours to digest a main meal), which means your 16-hour fast will end around 1 p.m. the next day.

Notice the shorter window of eating time. If you find this daunting at first, feel free to increase your fast time by an hour every day by moving your breakfast meal back until you feel more comfortable not eating breakfast. I'll share in a later chapter how fasting can benefit many of your hormones.

HGH Booster # 3: High Intensity Exercise

Intense exercise has also been shown to act as a natural human growth hormone stimulator. There are several theories why this occurs, but researchers agree that it seems to be in response to the breaking down of muscle. This includes resistance training and any other form of exercise that involves significant intensity.

It's true: regardless of the activity, it really is all in the intensity. No equipment is necessary.

So the best way to achieve this is with High Intensity Interval Training (HIIT).

HIIT involves alternating periods of high-intensity activity (sprints, circuit training, etc.) -with short periods of rest- for a total of 15 to 30 minutes of exercise. Beginners can start with just 10 minutes of total HIIT time, only 3 minutes of exercise time and still see nice results. So start small and work your way up.

A simple HIIT workout can include sprints, jump rope, cycling, rowing, and/or circuit training with or without weights. The key is to go *all out* in your effort during your "work" phase.

For instance, you do sprints at maximum effort for 30 seconds, then recover for 60 seconds, repeating for a total of 10, 15 or 30 minutes. Know that you can slowly increase the duration of your sprint time or decrease your rest time as you progress.

How to Truly Optimize HGH

Combining these three human growth hormone stimulators into your daily routine will have you naturally increasing your levels. However, depending on how imbalanced and depleted you are, time and commitment is required to see results. This is why in my clinic we like to employ the above lifestyle practices AND fast track the results using targeted supplementation and epigenetic modification.

Now You Can Age Optimally

I am so thrilled with the results our practice members have experienced as a result of befriending their youth hormone and implementing the four strategies into their lives.

CHAPTER 8:

The Sleep Hormone

S leep. It's one of the most important things we can do for our health, and yet research indicates that a huge number of people get less than seven hours of sleep each night especially moms of young children, the elderly and women over the age of 35. This has a lot to do with our "do-it-all" lifestyle that so many of us have adopted. But it's also a result of dysfunction in the body, genetic predispositions and imbalances in other hormones, all of which can be controlled and corrected.

Lack of sleep increases risk of cancer, heart disease, depression, weight gain, diabetes, brain fog, and simply not functioning well during the day. If you are not sleeping well, this book may help you identify the root cause and turn things around so you can start benefiting from hours of slumber each night.

Melatonin is the hormone we rely on to create our circadian rhythm (sleep-wake cycle) and give us the benefits of sleep.

It's amazing how our bodies respond to light and darkness. As the day comes to an end, our eyes pick up the change from light to darkness and send a signal to the pineal gland in the brain to start producing a hormone called melatonin. Each hormone communicates different messages within our bodies. Melatonin's main message is sleep. As melatonin levels increase and start circulating through our bodies, we become sleepy. As you might guess, melatonin levels are highest in the evening (around 10 pm) and are lowest during the daytime.

In addition to telling your body when it's time to sleep, melatonin is also an anti-oxidant and it influences your immune system and your mood. It's a clever hormone with a raft of possible benefits including:

63

- Helping with depression and Seasonal Affective Disorder (SAD)

- Pain Relief (such as with fibromyalgia)

- Preventing and even eliminating cancer cells

- Decreasing estrogen's influence on tumor growth, which is especially helpful in preventing breast cancer

- Knowing the benefits above helps us to understand why lack of sleep is so damaging

So, what causes melatonin to be low (when it should be high)? There are a number of things that influence melatonin production, including:

- Stress

- Lack of exposure to natural light during the day

- Exposure to blue light at night (often from television, phones, computers, and clocks)

- Working a night shift

- Travel and time zone changes (aka jet lag)

- Lack of sleep (i.e. parents up through the night with an infant/child)

- Intestinal permeability and nutrient deficiencies

If you're wondering if your melatonin is low, a dry urine test for comprehensive hormones (DUTCH) will give you a melatonin reading along with cortisol and your other steroid hormones. This is the best way to know, rather than simply guessing. Unfortunately, this test is not commonly done in a standard medical office or in sleep clinics, so you'll need to work with a naturopathic doctor (or functional medicine practitioner) who can do the test, interpret the results, and advise you on the support you need to get your melatonin levels back in balance.

Support and Treatment for Low Melatonin

Here are four simple things you can do if your melatonin levels are low that will help you get a good night's sleep:

Turn out the lights before 10 pm

Some sources even recommend turning down the lights at sunset or by 7 pm. I recommend that you dim the lights at least one hour before going to bed and, as much as possible, turn off electronic devices and other lights in your bedroom (even the smallest little light can lower your melatonin).

As I mentioned, melatonin is highest at bedtime, which is supposed to be at or before 10 pm. The later you stay up past that time, the less melatonin you will have, and the more difficult it will be to fall asleep.

Reduce exposure to blue light

If you must be exposed to lights after 10 pm, you can buy glasses that block blue light, the type of light that turns off melatonin production. There are many companies that make these glasses that stop the light from being noticed by your brain. You can also use special software on your computer to filter blue light and turn iPhone screens red to further protect yourself from the damaging blue light.

Check your serotonin levels

Melatonin is made in the body from tryptophan and serotonin. So if your melatonin is low, it is also important to consider whether your serotonin is low. Serotonin can be measured in a urine panel (if levels are low, they can be supported by taking a tryptophan or 5HTP supplement). As your serotonin levels increase, so will your melatonin levels. Often times, serotonin levels are low because of an issue in the gut or a genetic variation, both of which can be investigated and supported.

Take a melatonin supplement

You can take melatonin as a supplement* to help increase your levels. A common starting dose is 1 mg, taken within an hour of going to bed, optimally around 9 pm. If you don't see enough of a difference with 1 mg, you could increase to 2 or 3 mg, though I wouldn't advise doing this except on the advice of a qualified practitioner. You may also find that taking 1 to 5 mg of melatonin will help you adjust to a new time zone when traveling. I suggest taking the melatonin at bedtime (10 pm) in the new time zone. It is important to note that melatonin does not have addictive qualities or withdrawal symptoms, although it can cause your dreams to be more vivid.

* This approach is not the solution, but some relief care to allow you to get some sleep while investigating the reasons for low melatonin.

Digging Deeper

Melatonin, like other hormones, delivers important messages throughout your body. When it is low, often due to exposure to stress and light at night, we are likely to experience the negative effects of insufficient melatonin. It is such a valuable hormone in terms of sleep, as well as for healthy cells, immune function, and mood. So, it is worth identifying whether it is an issue for you and addressing it.

Now if you follow these steps and find that you are still not sleeping, then it's time to dig deeper and get a better understanding of what is keeping you awake. Quite often it is more than one thing. It could be that you have low melatonin and elevated cortisol, for example. Or perhaps it's a combination of leaky gut, food sensitivities, low serotonin, and low melatonin, all of which are related to each other, but need to be addressed individually to completely address your sleep issues. Or it could be that you have inflammation (whether from an injury or a food) that has disrupted your sleep.

To break these vicious cycles, we need to first understand all of the causes, and then address each of them in turn, using a systems-based approach. Then, little by little, over time, the body will start to adjust, and sleep will be restored. However, it's worth noting that it is often a process that requires patience and diligence, which can be challenging when you can't sleep.

CHAPTER 9:

How to Test Hormones

There are four main methods of testing for sex and adrenal hormones: Blood, Saliva, Wet Urine, and Dry Urine. They all have their own pros and cons.

Blood

Blood is the language of most physicians and is considered by many to be the worldwide gold standard. But in terms of cortisol, we only get one reading in the day, usually a morning reading. That's a big downside for blood testing, because when it comes to looking at the health of the HPA axis, we need to look at the up and down pattern of cortisol. The only way this would be possible is if you returned to the lab four times over the course of the day at a specific time.

Also, being stuck with a needle is stressful for some people. So, even if it was a good test for cortisol, it may not be a good test for everyone, because the anticipation of getting stuck with a needle can make your stress hormones go up.

The final downside of blood is that it does not show the metabolites of your hormones, such as estrogen, cortisol and testosterone, so we don't get as much information about how your hormones are behaving.

Blood testing for hormones, however, is usually covered by insurance, making it is a decent place to start.

Saliva

Salivary hormone testing has been the dominant model for sex and adrenal hormones in the alternative health world for at least 30 years. But there are some downsides. One downside is that it only shows the free fraction of cortisol, the cortisol that is not bound by a carrier protein. Thus, you will not see total cortisol and only get half of the picture.

Unfortunately, salivary hormone testing is not sensitive enough to test estradiol or any of the sex hormone metabolites. The final downside of salivary testing is that it can be difficult for some people to fill up two-inch vials with saliva. That is a lot of spitting!

The good thing about saliva is that it does capture the diurnal rhythm. Unlike blood, when using saliva testing you can capture the four-point rhythm byl testing throughout the day. So, saliva is a decent option, but it is somewhat incomplete and certainly not the best option.

24-Hour Urine

When doing a 24-hour urine test, you are collecting all of your urine in one big jug with no separation between your morning, noon and night samples. For that reason, this type of testing does not allow you to see the diurnal up and down pattern of cortisol.

This test can be a bit of a pain and the collection of that urine is somewhat cumbersome. You must collect every single drop of urine, otherwise, your test is invalid. One of the good things about a 24-hour urine test is that it can measure aldosterone. That's what some practitioners like to use for adrenal assessment. Another great thing about the 24-hour urine test is that it can measure metabolites of hormones.

Overall, 24-hour urine testing is decent, but not my top pick.

Dry Urine

This is a newer method of testing hormones and has only been around for a few years. The dried urine test combines the best aspects of saliva and 24-hour urine without the downsides. You get the four samples, allowing us to see the pattern of cortisol over 24 hours, and we can look at both free and bond forms of cortisol. And we can also examine the metabolites of our hormones, which is super-helpful in understanding how your hormones are

Section II

CHAPTER 10:

A Whole-Body Approach to Hormone Health

What I have found in my own experiences while working with thousands of women is that there's a real gap in our healthcare system. It is bro- ken. The way it's set up today is more a system of sick care than health care.

Here's how it works:

You start out pretty healthy: two eyes, two ears, one nose, a pumping heart and breathing lungs. All of your systems are functioning. You have a lot of vitality, the inner force that heals and keeps us energetic and strong. As you cruise through life, you come into contact with your environment, along with some stressors. As time goes on, there's physical stress, mental stress, biomechanical stress, all impacting and influencing your genetic and hormonal expression.

Your body has to deal with all the stress that comes in. So you're going along feeling good, but all the stress is coming at you. Maybe you have a sports injury. Perhaps your parents are fighting and you're dealing with some stress in your relationships. Maybe you get in trouble at school or you're eat- ing a whole bunch of candy and chips.

Eventually, with all these stressors acting upon you, you are bound to pick up a symptom here, a few symptoms there. Most of us will treat symp- toms with home remedies or over the counter drugs, just to get a little bit of the discomfort to go away.

As you get a little older, maybe you find yourself in a little bit more pain. You have some more despair and depression, and some of the symptoms are now getting unbearable. Those over the counter medications and home remedies, well, they're no longer working. This is the point where most of us go to the doctor.

We've all been there. You are feeling like crap, so you call the doctor and you get an appointment for two weeks down the road. The day arrives, and you show up at the doctor's office 15 minutes early, as per the instructions recited by the receptionist. Ninety minutes later, after you've read every article in the 6-year old Women's World Magazine and just began reaching for a war-torn edition of Reader's Digest, your name is called. You wait some more in the little room, tell your symptoms to the nurse and again to the doctor.

If you are lucky, the doctor will decide to run some tests. At this point you are going to end up with one of two scenarios.

Scenario One: Your doctor will choose a test based on your complaints. They'll say, "What seems to be the problem?" Then he's going to pick a test based on what you say. And maybe a diagnosis is found. If so, you'll be given a medication to help bring your lab test numbers back into the "normal" range. Often, you'll continue taking this medication for an indefinite amount of time. Chances are, you'll experience one or more side effects and you'll get an additional medication to control those new symptoms.

Scenario Two: The doctor runs that same test, but this time your numbers come back in the normal range. This means that you're not YET eligible for that medication to control your symptoms. In this case, the doctor will simply say "Let's keep an eye on it." He'll tell you to come back. You'll take that same test every 6 to 12 months. He'll check your numbers again and again until you get bad enough to qualify for that medication.

In other words, he is just waiting for you to get sick, so he can write you a prescription. The problem with both of these scenarios is that neither one includes a healing protocol. In other words, symptoms are just simply being looked at, and either suppressed or waiting to get worse. But there's no plan in place to restore your health.

In a nutshell, that is the problem with our modern medical system. Doctors are trained to treat symptoms and lab results, but not to truly address healing. It really is a sick care, disease care system. And I'm not just talking about conventional medicine. Many natural and alternative practitioners are just as guilty. Only instead of pharmaceutical drugs, these practitioners are prescribing natural supplements and herbal remedies to treat symptoms and their lab results.

I'm not against supplements. I'm not against herbal remedies. I actually use these daily in my practice. And guess what? I'm not even against prescription medications. I do feel that there is a time and a place for these types of pharmaceutical drugs and they have their place in medicine.

What I am against is simply suppressing symptoms without working towards identifying the root cause of the condition, and not putting a plan in place to help the body heal. I'm against just treating the symptoms and calling it a day. I think that it's a real disservice to any patient to not have a healing plan in place.

This is the gap that we really need to fill. Symptoms should not be looked at as something that just needs to be controlled with pills. Instead, they need to be understood for what they are. They're the body's way of telling us there's something wrong. It's a sign of dysfunction or disease in the body. In other words, symptoms are not the problem but the result of the problem. The real problem is dysfunction or disease within the body.

Before we talk about how to overcome your symptoms, how to harmonize your hormones naturally to get rid of dysfunction and disease, let's talk about what causes symptoms to happen in the first place.

The number one reason for hospital visits, doctors' visits, days missed from work, and the number one contributor to illness right now in this day and age is… drumroll please… STRESS.

Stress is your big enemy. Stress is what causes so many things to go wrong in your body. I mentioned earlier about how you start out your life full of vitality. You have lots of energy, and you're going about your life, but you're encountering little stressors along the way. You're encountering stressors that are mental, emotional, physical and biochemical.

As these stressors come into contact with your body. They influence your genetic and hormonal expression. However, although we tend to label stress as the bad guy, it's not always bad. I want you to know that there are two types of stress. There's distress, which is the stressors that we're going to talk about. These are the bad stressors that cause symptoms, that cause inflammation, that cause disease and dysfunction.

But there's also a good stress which gets us motivated. It turns on our brains and heightens our senses. It gets us to start and finish tasks and accomplish goals.

It's a stress that I used to have when I was on the college track team. At the beginning of each race, I waited on the starting line, shoulder to shoulder with the women I was about to battle. We waited with anticipation for the sound of a gunshot to signal the start of the race. Just the anticipation of what was about to go down started our hearts racing and adrenaline pumping. When the gun fired, we took off like cheetahs. The stress response - in this case, my heart racing and adrenaline pumping - was what helped me to compete. It can help you speak on stage, to meet a deadline, to introduce yourself in a crowd, ask for a raise. It is actually good stress. It is a stress that helps us act.

However, stress that contributes to dis-ease, that's what we call distress. The main problem for women in our modern world is that we condition ourselves to endure lots of stress. We ignore the body's signals that tells us that stress is too high, and instead "push through" or "suck it up", ignoring the fatigue, depression, anxiety, lowered immunity, hair loss, lack of libido, digestive distress, brain fog, and a host of other stress induced symptoms.

Mental/Emotional Stress: When we talk about stress -or your hear the word "stress"- what comes to mind for most people are the things that are "stressing them out".

Usually, it's things that have to do with relationships, money, health and the future... Pretty much anything that creates mental/emotional stress falls into one of those categories. Maybe you get stressed about your job, your mean boss or a deadline. Maybe you get stressed about your children eating their vegetables, or driving a car, or getting into college. Perhaps you stress about your health, your appearance, your weight or worry that you won't live to see your children get married and have children of their own. All of these thoughts create stress. This kind of stress originates in the mind.

The brain cannot differentiate between a danger or threat that you are facing right now, and one that you are imagining (aka worry). In other words, the same hormonal response occurs whether you are currently in danger or you are currently safe and sound but worrying. This is why chronic worry and chronic stress are so damaging to our hormonal balance and our health.

There are many ways to manage mental/emotional stress. You can do meditation, breathing exercises and reciting affirmations. Speaking to a friend, relative or therapist can also be helpful. Getting proper sleep, nutrition and movement can make you more resilient and better prepared to handle difficult situations calmly.

Physical stress: This type of stress can be easy to identify. It's the stress your body endures when you get an injury, have a surgery, give birth or get into an accident. It can be twisting your ankle, breaking a leg or getting into a major car accident. Anything that can cause trauma is a physical stress.

The other type of physical stress is the small tiny micro traumas that happen every day. Maybe you have a desk job where you sit at the desk, hunched over, staring at a computer screen and typing on a keyboard. Your eyes are being strained, your back is getting tight, your muscles are atrophying. That's a micro trauma, and over time, that competitive motion of typing, hunching over, the eye-strain, that's what we call physical stress in the body. It can show up as back pain, joint pain, bad eyesight, tight shoulders, weak muscles, brittle bones... and so on.

The problem could be your posture, it could be your shoes, it could be a job that you have. Maybe you're swinging your hammer, or you're typing, or you're carrying a serving tray. Whatever it may be, the major traumas and micro-traumas create stress in the body, which turns on our hormonal stress response.

Biochemical stress: This is the kind of stress that goes on without us really noticing. It's little chemical reactions that are happening in the body to create inflammation.

This can be exposure to toxins, mold in your home or the gasses that come off your carpeting and drapes from the flame-retardant chemicals. It could be toxins in your drinking water or in your air if you live near a factory or an auto repair shop. There're also things like food sensitivities, heavy metals, sugar, genetically modified foods, artificial flavors and colors, and for some people, even gluten and dairy. All of these things can contribute to stress in your body.

In our practice, we work on all three types of stress, but we focus on biochemical stress. After all, you're not going to go to physical therapy for biochemical stress. You're not going to go see a counselor or therapist for biochemical stress.

You really need a comprehensive systems-based holistic health-building plan to really deal with these biochemical stressors. It is important to first uncover what these biochemical stressors are, then remove the source of the stress and finally repair any damage that was done.

So, what does stress have to do with hormones?

Everything. Stress has everything to do with hormones and hormones have everything to do with overall health, happiness and longevity. So, stress is pretty significant. It is the missing piece when it comes to female hormone balance, especially for women over 35. Until the hidden biochemical stress is identified and removed, you will never feel truly balanced, even with all of the hormone replacement therapy in the world.

You will see exactly what I am talking about in the next chapter when I share my story about how I turned my personal pain into my purpose. But first, let's get into how symptoms actually come about in the body and how disease and dysfunction happen.

We all have a brain and a body that communicates back and forth using chemical messengers, also known as hormones. In a perfect scenario, everything is working correctly. Your heart, your lungs, your digestive system, your ovaries are all firing with 100% function, in a state of ease. This is what we refer to as "in balance." When all of your body's systems are working correctly, they have plenty of energy and no pain. This is an ideal situation and it is pretty much how most of us start out in life.

Case in point: toddlers. If you are a mom or have spent any time around children under the age of five, you know exactly where I am going with this. Toddlers rarely wake up in the morning with aches and pains. They can jump off park benches without worrying about hurting their knees. They have perfect squat form. And they seem to have an unlimited supply of energy. In fact, the entire time I have been writing this chapter, my three-year-old has been jumping up and down on the couch as if it were a trampoline.

Believe it or not, barring a few rare exceptions, we all once had that freedom from pain, optimized mobility, and seemingly endless energy. So, what happened? How did we get from there to here?

Stress. Stress happened.

As we grow up, we start to encounter all of these different stressors. Some mental/emotional stress, some physical stress and some biochemical stress all mashed up together. All of these stressors are interacting with your body. Genes are turned on and off, hormones go up and down, and symptoms occur. Maybe you experience pain, headaches, irritability, and some brain fog. Or maybe you have some diarrhea or constipation or some other issue.

When you have symptoms, what that means is that you're not at 100% function. The delicate balance has been thrown off and now you're at what we call dis-function or in a state of dis-ease.

So what's a girl to do? You might ignore the pain for a while, chalk it up to being a normal part of life. Maybe you take some over the counter medications, maybe some herbal remedies and supplements. Or -if it is really bad- then you might even go to the doctor for a prescription. In my world, this is what we call relief care.

Maybe the relief care eases your symptoms. This is an awesome thing, but unfortunately it can be confused with healing. You may take a few different things: something for your tummy, something for your joints, something for your brain. Easy-peasy and feeling great, right?

Here is the problem. While your symptoms are going away, you're not doing anything about the dis-ease, and you're not doing anything about the dis-function. There is no actual healing going on.

So, guess what happens? Symptoms start coming back. Sometimes you get the same symptoms you started with, but they also may come back in new places. This is because you still have dis-function and dis-ease, and when dysfunction and disease are left untreated, they get worse. Over time they compound.

You end up with all of these different symptoms, more than what you started with in the first place. So instead of just doing relief care, we're going to talk about a holistic systems-based approach to healing, and it's what I'm going to teach you about in this book.

With a holistic systems-based approach we identify what is actually causing the symptoms and remedy that. We're getting rid of symptoms, and we're also getting rid of disease. We're getting rid of dysfunction and you're going to get back to 100% function. That's why you don't just want to do relief care. That's why you really want a holistic systems-based approach to balancing hormones and optimizing health. In order to really heal and balance, you need an approach that figures out which stressors are causing your symptoms and actually get you to the point of healing.

One Size Does Not Fit All

Have you ever ordered a sweater from a catalog that was listed as "one size fits all", and then when the package arrived you quickly realized that there is no such thing?

Just take a look around. Go to Starbucks, the grocery store, church or the airport and you will see people come in all shapes and sizes, colors and flavors. Sure, we all have the same number of eyes, legs, fingers and toes, and our heads are all placed on top of our necks, but that does not make us the same.

So then why does medicine and science in general use such a one-size-fit-all approach? Why is it that everyone diagnosed with certain symptoms or conditions get the same treatment? (Put the blue peg in the blue hole). This is because genetically, we *do* all share between 99.5 and 99.9% identical DNA. All humans, in other words, have over 99% identical genes. When you look at it this way, it makes perfect scientific sense to treat everyone the same.

But what about that 0.1 to 0.5 percent? It may seem insignificant, but what you must consider is that the human genome is made up of three billion base pairs, which means 0.1% is still equal to three million base pairs.

In those three million differences lie the changes that give you red hair instead of blonde or brown eyes instead of blue. You can find changes that increase your risk of obesity or others that decrease your risk of heart disease; differences that make you taller or lactose intolerant or allow you to run faster.

Understanding your genetics gives you a template upon which to layer a systems-based approach to healing so it can be the most personalized, precise method of reaching your full potential.

CHAPTER 11:

Sick is not Normal

"Everything you need to heal, grow and thrive can be found within nature, the universe and within yourself"

- Dr. Michelle Sands

N ow that you have a little bit of an idea of how disease starts in the body, why symptoms occur, the types of stress that we encounter every day, and how these can be at the root of your symptoms, I want to share a little bit of my life with you. Even though we all come from different backgrounds and have different stresses, struggles and goals, I feel every woman can relate to this story.

It wasn't long ago that I felt hopeless and helpless. I wasn't sure that there was anything I could do to help myself. Like many of you, I accumulated a whole laundry list of symptoms in my younger years. Many of these, I just wrote off as simply the way things were. I suffered from acne, major digestive problems and painful periods. These had been the norm for me since junior high. I learned to suck it up and not complain. I remember my dad always told me, "Life sucks and then you die." What a horrible thing for a young girl to hear. I think I even started to believe it for a while.

It is sad to think about, but that statement holds true for many women who live each day with pain. It does suck, and many people believe that until they die.

I didn't realize this at the time, but I really wanted to prove my dad wrong. One of the problems in my family was that we just didn't talk about our problems. We didn't complain. If you were sick enough, you'd see a

81

doctor and get a pill to take care of whatever the problem was. And if you weren't sick enough, well then you just didn't complain about it.

As a child, I took a lot of antibiotics. My mom actually had a doctor friend who handed them out like candy on Halloween. Well not exactly, but he would send over a prescription just with a phone call. We didn't even have to go into the office. So at the first sign of a sniffle or a cough, my mom would give my brother and me antibiotics so we could get over the cold or the cough in no time.

By the age of 12, I was on birth control pills, not because I was sexually active, but to control my painful cycles. And I was taking antibiotics to control my acne. I was taking Tums like they were after dinner mints. Early in life, I learned to handle a lot of pain, both physical and emotional. My mom would comfort me with junk food.

Things started to change for me in the sixth grade. I was becoming more aware of my body and I knew I had to do something if I was ever going to get a Dean Randazzo (my middle school crush) to notice me.

I decided I was going to become a runner, so I started running on the cross-country team. Coach Shea, noticing that I wasn't like the other girls, took me under her wing and taught me about how food was actually fuel for my body, and how what I ate affected how I performed. She saw something in me that I could not see in myself and she spent extra time working on drills with me and correcting my form.

I hung on her every word; I was so interested in what she had to say. Maybe it's because she was so different from my family, a polar opposite of my mom. She was athletic, she was happy, and she joked around with us. She actually enjoyed life, and she told me that my body could do anything I wanted it to do. I just had to train it, feed it, and believe in it. Wow, that was completely revolutionary for me. It was such a deep contrast to my dad's "life sucks and then you die."

That's why I started learning as much as I could about physical fitness and nutrition. I did my best to implement what I learned despite the fact that there really wasn't any healthy food in our house. We followed the

Three P diet. Have you heard of it? It was pretty popular among low- er-middle class Italian families in New York in the 80's. Our diet consisted mostly of pizza, pasta and pastries. Rarely did a fruit or vegetable make an appearance at our dinner table. So if I wanted to be healthy, I was going to have to be creative.

I started by trading my lunches to other kids in my class. The lunch my mom packed was actually pretty much a kid's fantasy. I always had two cans of cola wrapped in tin foil (so they stayed cold until noon). There would be a bag of Doritos, some type of Hostess snack cake, typically a Twinkie or one of those cupcakes with the frosting squiggles on it. And then of course I had a bologna sandwich.

Now, the bologna sandwich wasn't a hit, but the sodas got traded for juice or milk. The Doritos would get me some carrots or celery sticks. The snack cake always got me a piece of fruit, usually an apple, orange or banana. I actually found a way to get a meal that would fuel my body for my sport and put me at the head of the pack of all of my races.

Fast-forward into college. All the hard work I put in while on the high school track landed me an athletic scholarship. I was working part-time as a personal trainer and studying for my nutrition certification, while at the same time double majoring in sports medicine and communications. From the outside looking in, I really had a charmed life. It was amazing. As a young student athlete on scholarship, at one of the most prestigious schools in the country, it looked like I had it all. But on the inside, I was struggling and falling apart. My digestive issues and period problems were wearing me down. Added to that, I started having joint pain and chronic fatigue. It had become unbearable trying to juggle everything, running track *and* dealing with my growing health issues.

That's when I began popping 5 or 6 Ibuprofens in the morning just to be able to walk to class. I basically lived on coffee, energy drinks, and diet coke all through the morning, then more ibuprofen before track practice. I'd have to wait until the late afternoon to eat so that my stomach wasn't hurting during my run.

I became dependent on laxatives to keep things moving in the morning, and it really turned into an endless process of popping a pill for a symptom. It was an extremely challenging time for me. When it came time for my annual athletic physical checkup, I decided to discuss everything that had been going on with me to the doctors. I actually broke down while in the clinic, telling them about some of my symptoms in more detail than they cared to hear. They agreed to run a few tests for me, and a few days later, I was delivered some life altering news.

The phone call I got that day was like a knife to my heart. But it was also a turning point in my health journey. Up until that point, I just accepted my symptoms as a normal part of life; bad genetics, perhaps. I did what I could to live a healthy lifestyle. I tried to eat fruits and vegetables. I got plenty of exercise running track. But in the end, I was dependent on Ibuprofen, over the counter medicines and caffeine to get me through my day. It was no way to live.

I'll tell you about this phone call with my doctor in just a minute, but first I want to point out a few of the things - a few of the myths - that I believed about health early in my life; myths maybe you were taught to believe as well. I've found that these beliefs are pretty common among the women I speak with, coming from what we've been told by society, causing us to simply accept them as truth.

Myth #1: Symptoms are Normal

Just because something is common, doesn't mean that it's normal. Eight out of ten people experience back pain; therefore, you could say that back pain is common. However, that does not mean that it is normal to have a painful back.

If you go to your local pharmacy or the supermarket, there are entire aisles dedicated to over-the-counter remedies for digestive issues like constipation, diarrhea, heartburn and nausea. Digestive issues are very common. In fact, Americans alone spend more than 2.2 billion dollars on antacids every year. That's a lot of heartburn. It's common to feel like crap after you eat, but that doesn't make it normal. As I mentioned before, symptoms are just a result of dysfunction in the body.

Myth #2: If your lab results come back normal, there is nothing wrong

This is really deceiving. If you've ever looked at your lab tests (I mean really looked), then you're familiar with the little reference ranges written down the side. In conventional medicine, if your numbers fall within that reference range, then you're considered fine, which really means that your problems aren't treatable with drugs or surgery.

There are a few problems with this way of medicine. First, the reference ranges are similar to grading a test on a curve. They take out the highest score and the lowest score, and then they get a middle average of all the people that took the test. The problem with this is that most of the time people who are taking lab tests for specific symptoms are doing so *because* they're experiencing symptoms. Therefore, what you end up with is a reference range that's the average of all the sick people. Now mind you, this isn't the case for every marker, but it is especially true for hormones, inflammation and other markers of performance and longevity.

In our clinic, we use optimal ranges instead of reference ranges. Optimal ranges are actually much narrower and include a much smaller spectrum of what's considered to be optimal. These numbers reflect healthy individuals with no symptoms or dysfunction.

Another problem with relying solely on lab tests is sometimes symptoms are a spillover from the dysfunctions in other areas of the body. We talked about this earlier, and you're limited by the lab tests you choose to run, so when symptoms are present, it's important to keep digging, even after one or two lab tests come back looking "fine."

If the tests come back within range, then the issue or dysfunction is likely in an unrelated system. So, if you're having symptoms, any symptoms, remember that although it may be common, that it's not normal, and you need to keep digging for answers.

Lisa's Story

One of my patients, Lisa, was experiencing the following symptoms: she was dealing with weight gain and couldn't maintain a healthy weight no matter what she did. She had low energy, constant fatigue, her hands and feet were cold all of the time, her skin was dry, she was losing hair, she was having difficulty sleeping, she had some muscle aches, constipation, and swelling in her ankles.

On top of that, she felt depressed. All of these symptoms together, if you speak to any medical professional, are classic signs of thyroid dysfunction. I wouldn't even need a lab test to tell you that. But Lisa went to her primary care doctor and he tested her TSH (Thyroid-Stimulating Hormone), which came back normal. It was tested six months prior, and while it climbed a few points over that period, the numbers still came back in the normal range. Although her numbers were trending up, they were still in the normal range.

So, Lisa was sent away and told to relax, that she was normal and nothing was wrong. She was actually offered an antidepressant and some pain pills for her muscle pain. Luckily, Lisa knew deep down something was wrong. As luck would have it, while searching the internet for answers, she happened upon one of my videos where I was talking about thyroid dysfunction and secondary thyroid dysfunction. I explained that with secondary thyroid dysfunction, your lab tests might come back normal, but you still have thyroid issues. Lisa contacted me immediately and we began working together. Within a month, we uncovered that she had a good deal of dysfunction in her digestive and immune system. Her thyroid was not the primary issue, even though her symptoms appeared to be thyroid related, they were actually related to different systems in the body, which we were then able to address.

The moral of the story is that even if your doctor tells you your test results are normal, and you're still experiencing symptoms, further investigation is needed.

Myth # 3: Your Genes Determine Your Destiny

This is one I hear all of the time and used to believe it myself. Many people believe that our genes determine our fate and that we're doomed to certain illnesses if it runs in our family. This really could not be further from the truth. Aside from a very small segment of the population - less than 2% of people are born with irreversible genetic defects - the other 98% of us have the power to control our genetic expression. It's really quite empowering. The latest research confirms that every action we take, from what we think to what we eat, to how we move, to where we live, all affect our genetic expression. This is called Epigenetics. You now have the power to leverage your genetics in order to optimize your health. Our practice members can now create precise bio individual lifestyle plans that optimizes their health faster and with less guess work.

The big takeaway is that you're not doomed to have the same diseases that your parents had. You *do* have the power to change. Sure, there are tendencies and predispositions that can be handed down through time, but ultimately, our lifestyle, our environment, and our mindset determine how those genes are expressed.

Myth # 4: Getting Healthy is Hard

This is a huge myth, because the reality is that being sick is a lot harder. Living in pain is hard. Being overweight, depressed or suffering from any of the conditions that we talked about early is certainly harder than eating healthy, living well, sleeping well, taking care of ourselves, and exercising. All of those things are far less painful than pain itself (and far less expensive too). If you add up all of the money that you're spending on over the counter remedies, supplements, doctor appointments and prescriptions, you could save yourself a ton of money and a ton of heartache if you just worked on improving your health.

I understand that some of us have felt bad for so long that we kind of forget and lose sight of what it's like to actually feel good. I remember those early college years when I was barely getting by. I actually thought I was fine because I'd been dealing with the symptoms for so long that they just be-

87

came a part of my life. It was what I knew; it was my identity. But let me tell you, once I started really healing... Wow! It was like I was totally reborn. And a whole new world opened up for me, which brings me back to my story...

I left you hanging there. I told you about how I went for my annual athlete physical exam and I broke down and told the doctor what I'd been dealing with, all of the pain and discomfort that I was going through. Several days after that appointment, I got the call that changed the course of my entire life. I was on the phone with a girlfriend at the time and we were talking about our plans for the weekend (I think there was some party on campus we wanted to go to), and the phone beeped, letting me know there was a call on the other line.

I thought it was my date calling to let me know our plans for dinner, but it wasn't. Instead, it was the clinic. Dr. Silva had my test results.

First, the "good" news. He said, "You don't have any major digestive issues. Your test results came back normal".

Glancing across my dorm room at the stockpile of antacids and laxatives, I thought, *normal?* I hesitantly replied, "Cool, thanks..."

I was ready to hang up the phone, but Dr. Silva continued, driving a stake through my heart. He explained that my hormone levels were significantly depressed, and that my ovaries were not working. They had failed. Because of the severity of the issue, he told me that I would never be able to have children and likely have lifelong issues of bone loss and depression, which he could give me a prescription for.

This was extremely difficult for me to hear. I had just been sucker punched in the stomach. I couldn't breathe and words wouldn't form. My heart raced, beating uncontrollably, and my palms pooled beads of sweat. If I weren't frozen in disbelief, I would have sobbed. I held the phone in my hand, listening to silence. The doctor broke the silence by offering antidepressants and anti-inflammatories, but not much else, and certainly not answers. Still unable to speak, I hung up the phone, afterwards staring at the ceiling for an hour, maybe two. I didn't know what I was going to do.

I sulked for a while after, a long while - a couple of years, actually. And I didn't tell anybody about what was going on with me. I felt like if I ignored it, maybe it would go away. Like a child hiding from the boogeyman under her sheets, if I hid from this, maybe it too would go away. But it didn't. Every year on Mother's Day I would sink into a horrible depression thinking about what could have been. I looked around at all of the moms, the healthy moms, playing with their children, and I knew that would never be me.

Three years later, on Mother's Day, I decided to stop feeling sorry for myself and to get answers. I thought about what my track coach had told me in sixth grade, that my body could do anything I wanted it to do, that I just had to train it, feed it, and believe in it.

My healing journey began that day. And it wasn't linear. I actually made lots of mistakes. My focus was strictly limited to healing my hormones, since I was trying to treat my symptoms and my lab results.

I tried bio-identical hormones, herbs, supplements, and acupuncture. I pretty much tried any treatment that anybody would offer me, or anything I could find. I just really wanted to get better. Some of my symptoms did improve, but they would always come back. I felt like I was taking one step forward and two steps back, which frustrated me to no end.

I then decided to go back to school and study Naturopathic Medicine, becoming my own a human lab rat. I ran every test and every protocol that I learned about on myself.

Then I made a shocking discover that completely changed my focus. What I found was both devastating and empowering. Not one, but two diseases that had gone undiagnosed for the majority of my life were holding me back and keeping me from healing. So, now I had a new problem to solve, a new area of focus.

CHAPTER 12:

From a Whole List of Symptoms to a Holistic Solution - The Five Step Plan

f I was really going to heal and achieve balance, there could be no more guessing, no more trial and error, no more half-assing the process, I had to go about this in a systematic and scientific way. Looking back on my journey, I can describe the entire healing process into five distinct steps.

Step 1: Define and Declare

I started by getting clear on what I wanted. I had learned from running long distance that if you don't set a specific finish line or you don't know where it is, you will likely stop short of your goal when things start to get uncomfortable. One thing that I wanted above anything was to be a mom. That was evident to me when I was only a child and had unwrapped my first baby-doll. I wanted to hold that baby in my arms tightly.

I also wanted more energy. I wanted smooth digestion, clear skin and freedom from pain. Those were the things that I defined and declared for myself as a must have. Those were my non-negotiables. I promised myself I would not stop fighting until every one of these goals became my reality, no matter how bumpy the road.

Step 2: Identify and Remove Blocks to Health

I took a long hard look at my life. I analyzed my own eating, sleeping and exercise routines. I took note of the things that caused stress in my life. I examined my relationships, my faith and my negative self-talk. I looked for any and every possible link to my imbalances.

As a medical student and nutritionist, I had access to some really interesting lab tests. Being the adventurer that I was, I started running every lab that I could get my hands on. That's when I discovered many imbalances. It's also when I realized that I actually had two diseases, likely from a very young age, that were preventing me from healing my hormones.

All the work I had previously done, all the bio-identical hormones, special diets and supplements, all these things I had been doing weren't really working. Or at least they weren't working in the long term because of both diseases. I had Celiac disease, which is an autoimmune condition, and Hashimoto's Thyroiditis, another autoimmune condition.

An autoimmune condition is basically where your body is attacking itself. In Hashimoto's Thyroiditis, it actually starts attacking your thyroid. And with Celiac Disease, it actually starts attacking your gut lining. Celiac Disease is a true intolerance to gluten where your body is looking at that gluten molecule and mistaking it for your own body's tissue.

As an Italian girl growing up in New York, where we basically ate pizza and pasta and bread all of the time, that was not a good thing for me. This new information really changed my life. I eliminated gluten and I stopped having the horrible digestive problems. Although I still had some, finding this out made a world of difference for me.

Hashimoto's, on the other hand, was a little trickier. Not many practitioners knew how to handle it back then. I was told by natural medicine doctors, alternative medicine doctors and conventional medical doctors that there was no cure for Hashimoto's. So I would basically be on medication for the rest of my life. I took the medication and accepted the life-sentence to medication. In the back of my mind, I knew one day I would overcome this as well. I put myself on a specific diet, changed the way I exercised, changed how I slept, and lowered my stress load. And I took some herbal extracts and supplements to support healing. Eventually, my antibodies went down to nearly nothing.

I also had what's called leaky gut, where molecules from your intestines start leaking into your bloodstream, so I had to do a whole gut repair protocol to heal my gut. I also ended up having a parasite. Being that my microbiome was compromised, I would travel or simply go out to eat and I would get sick. Meanwhile, my friends, who had a healthy microbiome, felt fine.

That's why sometimes two people can go eat at the same restaurant and one person will get sick and the other person will be like, "No, it must not have been the food because I'm fine." Well the person with the compromised microbiome or gut lining is more likely to get sick because they have that hospitable environment for those pathogens to come in.

Bottom line: I had to do a lot of work identifying and removing pathogens, yeasts, immune responders, and food allergies that were really hurting me, so that was what I did. I had to make changes to my lifestyle in order for healing to happen.

Step 3: Nourish and Support

This step is really important. I had to heal my gut. I had to heal my microbiome. I had to both calm and boost my immune system and I had to restore the healthy function of my thyroid, adrenals and ovaries. That took some work, some patience, and a whole lot of TLC. I committed strict adherence to a diet of nourishing foods, supplements and also changed the way I thought and the way I exercised.

I had always been one of those Type A personalities. I always had to win. I always had to be first. I always had to get an A+. Learning to enjoy the moment and be more present, learning that I didn't always have to be first or the best, and learning how to take it easy on myself really helped support my body in healing. After all, that mental/emotional stress I was putting on myself was preventing my body from being healing.

I had to stop running long distance marathons and eating such a low-fat diet, since that was putting too much stress on my body and not giving it the building blocks it needed to support my hormones. Remember, your hormones are made out of cholesterol. I had to change my diet to include healthy fats and organic proteins. I had to nourish my body so that it could actually create those building blocks to heal itself.

Step 4: Balance

Notice this is Step 4, not Step 1. The problem with many healing protocols is that balance is put too early in the process. This is why so many women are taking hormones and still feel like crap.

Think about it this way: Imagine that your house is on fire. You attempt to put it out by spraying it with your garden hose. Just when you appear to be making some progress, the flame kicks up again. What you don't realize is that there is an arsonist on the other side of your house pouring fuel on the fire. Until the arsonist is removed, your efforts will be futile.

The same is true with balancing hormones. You really need to take the time to identify what it causes the imbalance and remove or correct that. Then nourish and support the body to regain homeostasis. Only once that is accomplished can you truly balance. This is precisely why I had such a hard time in the early years of my health journey; I was trying to balance first.

Once you have identified and removed the majority of the sources of your dysfunction, you can concentrate on balance. This is when you can start dialing things in, start balancing hormones, balancing neurotransmitters and balancing the microbiome, and creating balance in your life. Rest and activity, fun and work, wake and sleep, good and bad, everything must balance.

Once I felt balanced, I realized I was ready to have a child. Despite what I had been led to believe most of my life, I became pregnant and I had my son Paxton, the most amazing child in the world.

That was when I knew I had won. I was told it would never happen, that there was no hope for me, that the best I could do was take some pills to dull the pain. When I first laid eyes on Paxton, I knew that I had to share this approach with other women, with all women. Whether their goal was to become a mom, or to lose 50 lbs, to get off a medication, reverse diabetes, clear up their skin, break free from pain or live a longer more vital life, this was the system that would help them. I started working with a small group of women, taking them through the steps, and the results were shocking.

Every woman saw improvements in their health and their confidence. Since then, this system has come to be known as The GLOW Protocol and has helped thousands of women.

Step 5: Thrive, Optimize and Enhance

There is one more step in the system. It is to take your body and mind to the next level, thrive and optimize. This is what I'm still doing now, and I think that it's important to note that you're never really done. This is the next stage in human evolution. This is what makes GLOW different. Conventional medicine is about preventing death and managing disease. Functional Medicine is about bringing your body back into homeostasis. My goal for you is to go beyond neutral, beyond balance, to a newly elevated state of optimal wellness.

I'm in my 40s now. So as I get older, I want to make sure that I really set myself up for healthy aging and for a long, healthy, active life. It's important to note that you need to go through the first four steps first. And sometimes life may throw you a curve ball and you might have to go back through the process. That is okay, because you will continue to evolve with each step. What's important is that you don't give up on yourself. Joy, happiness, balance, and in my case, Paxton, is all worth it. What do you have to lose? Your pain?

CHAPTER 13:

Identity Crisis

Now that you know my story and why I am writing this book, I want to share with you the story of one of my patients. Her name is Janey, an amazing woman. She was a personal trainer who enjoyed instructing hip-hop aerobics. I had actually seen videos of her a few years prior to meeting her, where she was doing these crazy acrobatics on stage.

When I first met Janey, she wasn't doing acrobatics on stage any more nor teaching classes. She wasn't even able to go to the gym since she had no energy at all. The worst part was that she was starting to gain weight. If you looked at her, if you met Janey when I met her, you wouldn't be like, "Oh that Janey, she's so fat!" You wouldn't even think that she was overweight at all. For Janey, however, her profession, her career, her passion was being a role model for physical fitness. For her to start losing muscle tone and gaining belly fat was really devastating. She had no energy to even workout with her clients. Eventually, she had to take a leave of absence from working at the gym.

It was really devastating for her because that's really what her passion was. And for her not to be able to fulfill her passion really brought her down. Her moods were low. She was having difficulties in her relationship with her husband since she no longer felt like herself.

We went through the steps, starting with defining and declaring what she wanted. What she wanted was to get back to her ideal weight and have her old energy back. We went through her current state of health, including a detailed questionnaire and system specific assessments. It wasn't long before I started uncovering that she had a bunch of other symptoms, which weren't at the forefront of her mind because she was so focused on her main goal, which was physical fitness and energy.

Through the assessments, I found a lot of digestive issues. She also had cold hands and feet, along with a little bit of hair loss, a low libido, among several other issues.

We ran a battery of tests. We did an endocrine test, which measured all of her hormones and a complete thyroid test. We also did a comprehensive microbiome and gut health test. The gut test revealed that she wiped out of all the good bacteria and she had a buildup of bad bacteria. These bacterial imbalances were hurting her energy production. As well, her imbalanced gut was throwing off her hormone balance and blocking the conversion of her thyroid hormones.

In this case, her thyroid organ was doing the work it needed to do, so that wasn't the problem. The problem was the conversion from inactive thyroid hormone to the active thyroid hormone because much of this happens in your gut (20%). Because this wasn't happening, it was draining her energy.

She had a very healthy diet. But because that she didn't have the proper balance in her microbiome, she wasn't able to actually absorb and assimilate the nutrients. In other words, she could not properly extract the nutrients out of the food and bring it to herself and her body. So that caused the mood issues, fatigue and loss of muscle.

We identified those issues and we started removing them systematically. We started nourishing Janey's body with some restorative, regenerative, easy to assimilate foods and supplements. We then went step-by-step, building her strength back, building her confidence back and taking some time to teach her how to not be so hard on herself.

We were supporting her not only in her mental and emotional state, her energy level, her confidence and her perspective, but we were also supporting all of the systems within her body so that she could heal efficiently and reach a 100% state of function.

While the main focus was on her energy and her strength, we were actually working on her thyroid and her hormones, her gut, and all the organs that produce energy, allowing for muscle building and fat loss. We were also working on detoxification, circulation and transport as well as cellular membranes and immune response. Everything mentioned above was necessary to help her support her body in healing itself on a holistic level.

We worked on balancing her hormones and really getting them to an optimal state, not just in the normal range for her age, but at the upper end of the normal range where she's actually going to feel amazing. We worked on balancing her neurotransmitters since, often when there's a hormonal imbalance, there's also a neurotransmitter imbalance. So we gave her some support there. And then we balanced her microbiome, which is definitely important when there are any GI issues and any immune issues.

Getting all of those things into balance allowed her to get back into the gym, start getting back to her ideal weight, her ideal body type, and enjoying her life and having energy again. Her sex drive came back as well as improvements in her relationship with her husband.

Janey didn't stop there. She went on to thrive and optimize. She's now really passionate about helping other people reach their optimal level of fitness and is now a role model for midlife women.

CHAPTER 14:

The Gut Hormone Connection

You may have heard the saying, "All disease begins in the gut." I am not sure I agree with it 100%. After all, you have to be at least a bit skeptical of any claims that include the words "always', "all", and "every." I do, however, believe that gut health affects nearly all other areas of health, hormones included.

Almost every one of the women I have worked with over the past decade has had some level of gut dysfunction, contributing to hormonal imbalances.

If you are wishing to balance your hormones, a good place to start is with the gut. Poor gut health nearly always leads to suboptimal hormone health.

How Your Gut Can Negatively Affect Your Hormone Health

Hunger and Cravings

The hormones that control your appetite are affected when your gut is unhealthy because it promotes the growth of unhealthy bacteria. This imbalance between good bacteria and bad bacteria alters the levels of ghrelin and leptin. Ghrelin is like an alarm that rings every time you're hungry and it's time to eat. Leptin lets you know you're full and it's time to put the fork down. Interestingly, an imbalance between healthy and unhealthy bacteria in your gut also affects which foods you crave and what foods you enjoy eating. So in all likelihood, those uncontrollable cravings are more about your microbiome than your motivation.

Mood and Sleep

Did you know that around 80% of serotonin and melatonin in your body are made in your gut? An imbalance in serotonin (the happiness hormone) and melatonin (which optimizes sleep) get completely out of whack when you have Irritable Bowel Syndrome (IBS), Leaky Gut Syndrome or other complications with your digestive tract. An imbalance in the hormones directly responsible for your happiness and quality of sleep may result in feelings of depression, anxiety, trouble sleeping and more.

Stress and Cortisol

Suffering from leaky gut syndrome or irritable bowel syndrome (IBS) also causes your inflamed gut to create an increased stress response in your body. You become easily stressed, increasing cortisol levels. Many studies have shown that taking probiotics daily can lower your cortisol levels and reduce your stress response.

Estrogen Dominance

When your gut health is off, so are your Estrogen levels. When you suffer from IBS or leaky gut syndrome it's impossible for your body to effectively remove estrogen from your body and keeping it in circulation, which causes Estrogen Dominance. A dominance in estrogen causes an imbalance of estrogen and progesterone, which needs to be in perfect balance in order for your body to properly support menstrual functions, promote fat burning and lower fluid retention. Estrogen dominance also alters your weight, stress levels, sleep patterns, appetite and slows your metabolism.

Thyroid and Metabolism

If your gut is unhealthy, your body's ability to convert the T4 thyroid hormone into the more effective T3 form is compromised because this function occurs in your gut. This explains why many women with digestive issues that take Synthroid, a synthetic type of the T4 hormone, often do not feel well because they have issues converting it into T3.

Additionally, diseases such as hyperthyroidism, caused by an imbalance in the thyroid, can result in symptoms such as anxiety, thinning of the hair, slowed metabolism, irregular periods, sporadic weight loss or weight gain, insomnia and more. Leaky gut and inflammation can lead to autoimmune thyroid issues and those are often made worse by eating certain foods, such as gluten.

Blood Sugar

Your blood glucose level is also directly related to the health of your digestive tract. The healthier your gut is, the more stable your blood glucose level, the less sugar and sweets you crave, and the less insulin you release. Inversely, an unhealthy gut can create an insulin resistance, lowering your body's fat burning ability. Unsurprisingly, an unhealthy gut can also be to blame for diabetes, vision loss, fatigue, weight gain, skin problems, etc.

Well then, WHY, with all this information, is the gut a totally overlooked area when women are dealing with obvious hormonal issues?

Unfortunately, doctors, health experts, and even the women themselves are focusing on the endocrine system of the body. They look for problems with the various glands: thyroid gland, adrenal glands and reproductive glands. They are taking hormones, supplements and adaptogens and things that can affect hormone balancing within the body. If you read my story, this is exactly what I did for many years before I understood the importance of a systems-based approach.

Often, the entire endocrine system within the microbiome is largely ignored. Yes, that's right. The microbiome is now considered to be an endocrine organ. It is as powerful, if not, in some respects, more powerful than all of your other endocrine organs combined: your thyroid, pancreas, adrenal glands and your ovaries.

What is clear now, from all of the most recent studies, is that the microbiome produces and secretes virtually every hormone that the body utilizes. It also regulates the expression of these hormones and it can inhibit or

100

enhance the production of certain hormones in the body. So the microbiome plays a central, almost a controlling role, in what happens to hormone balance.

If you're dealing with hormone imbalances and you don't address the gut and the microbiome, you really won't get very far in getting those hormones balanced. We're fortunate that there's now plenty of studies showing us what is happening with the gut in respect to hormone balancing.

Maybe you've heard that serotonin is largely produced in the gut. Well, most researchers are supporting this data, that almost 90% of serotonin is made in the digestive tract. Serotonin is actually a master regulator of the communication between the gut and the brain. It is known as the happy hormone and it alters mood. It also alters things like your ability to sleep and relax, gut motility, and how well food moves through your digestive system. So a lot of times, indigestion, constipation, all of these things can be a factor of low serotonin. That can then spiral into mood and sleep issues as well.

Depression can certainly start in the gut. It can be triggered by something as simple as antibiotics. Even taking a course of antibiotics for something super common, like a sinus infection, can disrupt the microbiome. This disruption can send you into that downward spiral of low serotonin, dopamine, and thyroid hormone, which turns on a whole anxiety cascade. The gut produces things like dopamine, which is extremely important for reward centers of the brain and for making you feel happy. If you don't have enough dopamine, it's very hard to get satisfaction from the things you do. This is where addictions come in. You can easily develop a chemical dependency on that reward, and the body requires that chemical reward in order to motivate you to do things.

Low dopamine can also trigger increases in stress hormones, which lead to inflammation and more depression and anxiety.

A balanced microbiome is also very important for maintaining optimal estrogen levels, especially as we head into perimenopause and menopause.

We have three forms of estrogen in the body: Estrone, estradiol and estriol. Of course they each have different purposes. What you might not realize is that the microbiome actually produces all of these. It's not just your ovaries that make estrogen; your gut does too.

A healthy microbiome will produce more estriol than any of the other two versions. The benefit of estriol, which is often ignored in medical literature because it is the weakest of all of the estrogens, is that estriol can be protective.

Estriol used to be thought of as the pregnant woman's estrogen, and it was believed that that was all it was good for, since it was so weak. Estriol has this great capability to be weak, meaning it doesn't induce the estrogen dependent cancer and imbalance issues. Yet it gives you the all benefits of estrogen, like reducing menopausal symptoms, reducing vaginal dryness and reducing osteoporosis.

Low levels of estriol are correlated with higher degrees of bone loss. What women over 35 really need is for the microbiome to produce more estriol so that you don't end up having an elevation of estrone. In fact, there's a lot of research going on right now in breast cancer regarding how to increase Estriol levels naturally.

Another role of the microbiome is, in addition to making estrogens, it also helps to clear estrogen from the system. Breaking down and metabolizing estrogen is important to avoid estrogen dominance and all of the unfavorable symptoms that are associated with it. The estrobolome is a collection of enzymes that are produced by microbes within the gut whose job it is to break down estrogen and metabolize it, which is one of the main ways your body clears estrogen, using the microbiome.

So you can see, when it comes to balancing hormones, the gut is one of the key places to focus.

CHAPTER 15:

Hormones vs. Your Brain, Who's in Charge?

T hanks to advances in modern medicine, we are living longer than past generations. We're also finding that living longer does not necessarily bring happiness since "quality of life" depends on being healthy and balanced.

For many people, their greatest fear is losing their mind or memory as they age. The good news is that current research indicates that with balanced hormones, we can effectively improve brain health, even in our later years.

How the Brain Works

The brain is the most fascinating and least understood organ in the entire body. There is much we don't know about how the brain works, but a basic understanding of what we do know is necessary to discuss brain health.

The components that make up the brain consist of trillions of nerve cells called neurons. Each neuron has branch-like tentacles, called dendrites, for receiving information, along with a tail-like tentacle, called an axon, for sending information. The dendrites and axon of one neuron reaches over to, but does not quite touch, other neurons. The gaps or spaces between the neurons are called synapses. Each neuron has many dendrites and synapses, providing a huge number of potential connections.

Brain cells communicate with each other by releasing hormones, called neurotransmitters, which travel over the synapses to relay information between brain cells. Neurotransmitters relay every thought and feeling we experience. Neurotransmission is the scientific name for the brain processes that determine how we think, feel, behave and how we function.

Researchers know that there are many different kinds of neurotransmitters, but have identified only about 50 of them so far. Some of the most common are acetylcholine, adrenaline (epinephrine), noradrenaline (norepinephrine), dopamine, serotonin, glutamate and GABA. These chemicals "either excite or depress the cells they reach." They exist in an intricate balance constantly being released and broken down.

The different parts of the brain produce different types of neurotransmitters and in turn, also respond differently to the various neurotransmitters depending on a variety of factors.

For example, neurotransmission can be weak or strong, depending on the quantity and quality of neurotransmitter molecules, how well those molecules bind to their receptors, and whether or not there are enough receptors present. Current research indicates that each of these factors is affected by diet, exercise, hydration, and hormone balance.

Deteriorating brain health is usually diagnosed based on problems with cognition or memory.

Dementia (sometimes referred to as senility) is the gradual deterioration of cognition such that it interferes with daily living. It is caused by diseases that affect the brain and is not necessarily the outcome of aging. Dementia can influence all aspects of the mind and behavior, including memory, judgment, language, concentration, visual perception, temperament, and social interactions.

Memory loss is one of the most common complaints and fears of aging. As we age, we typically need more time to remember things, and our ability to concentrate tends to diminish. This is called Mild Cognitive Impairment (MCI), and can be exacerbated by poor nutrition, dehydration, and hormone imbalances, among other things. Even though MCI is "normal" and may not seriously affect daily living, there is some evidence that people with MCI over the age of 65 are likely to develop Alzheimer's disease within five years. However, most experts agree that Alzheimer's is a distinct disease and not necessarily the inevitable end result of the normal aging process.

Hormone Balance and Brain Health

Women going through menopause often feel like they're losing their minds. A hormone imbalance can wreak havoc on brain chemistry and communication between brain cells. Estrogen, progesterone, testosterone, and thyroid hormones are as essential to our moods and cognitive ability as nutrients are to our basic cellular function.

In fact, concentrations of the estrogens, progesterone, pregnenolone, testosterone, DHEA and other hormones can be higher in the brain than in the bloodstream. Research indicates that nerve cells in the brain (and central nervous system) are actually producing their own supply of these hormones, independently of hormone production by the ovaries, testes and adrenal glands.

Because hormones are often more concentrated in the brain, any hormone imbalance can affect brain function dramatically. Deficiencies in cortisol, DHEA, estrogen hormones, melatonin, pregnenolone, testosterone, thyroid, and vasopressin exhibit the most common brain-related symptoms, including memory loss, poor concentration, and confusion.

Chronic medical conditions, especially those linked with a hormone imbalance, typically also have a profound impact on brain health and often lead to memory problems. Conditions commonly associated with memory loss are depression, arteriosclerosis, blood sugar problems, chronic fatigue syndrome, fibromyalgia, allergies, and infections such as candida, all of which are often associated with hormone imbalance.

Specific hormones and their effects on the brain

Estrogens

The estrogen hormones - primarily estrone, estradiol (the most abundant) and estriol - offer significant health benefits for women. These estrogens have profound effects on brain health in both men and women including:

- Promoting networking between brain cells by increasing the number of dendritic branches

105

- Increasing levels of the mood-regulating neurotransmitters, including acetylcholine, serotonin, and noradrenaline
- Increasing the density of neurotransmitter receptors
- Maintaining nerve cell health by encouraging nerve growth and preventing the accumulation of free radicals
- Helping to prevent brain damage by reducing inflammation and promoting brain cell repair when damage occurs
- Promoting brain vibrancy by increasing blood flow to the brain, which increases the oxygen and glucose available

Testosterone

Certain hormones, such as testosterone, may also influence our ability to perform different types of thinking tasks. Studies have shown that men and women who have better spatial memory (which allows precise movements in space, such as handling tools or dancing) have higher levels of testosterone than their peers. Women who excel in mathematics have also been found to have high testosterone levels.

In both men and women, testosterone strengthens muscles, arteries, and nerves, including those in the brain (although it has a more profound effect in men, whereas estrogen has a more profound effect in women). Without enough testosterone, the arteries in the brain weaken, growing too soft in some places - increasing the risk of blood clots and stroke - and too stiff in others - increasing the risk of high blood pressure and cerebral hemorrhage - none of which is good for the memory. When the arteries of the brain wear out, blood can no longer properly circulate to the brain or to any other organ for that matter. When the resulting lack of oxygen and nutrients to the brain is chronic, memory weakens. As well, human growth hormones work in concert with testosterone to keep neural arteries strong.

Thyroid

Thyroid hormones also have significant effects on thought processes and memory. In the brain's gray matter, where thinking takes place, the blood begins to flow more slowly as thyroid levels decline. As a result, less oxygen and fewer nutrients reach the brain cells, the brain becomes malnourished, causing you to think and moves less. Without enough thyroid hormones, the number of connections (dendrites and synapses) between the brain cells decrease, weakening the brain cells.

Fortunately, this process can be reversed with proper treatment.

Pregnenolone

This is often referred to as "the memory hormone" because of its astounding ability to improve memory. Research has shown that pregnenolone works as a neurotransmitter to clarify thinking, promote concentration, and prevent memory loss. One of its more unusual effects, according to some women, is that it seems to intensify color perception.

Pregnenolone is the most abundant hormone in the brain and is concentrated about 75 times greater in the brain than in the blood. It serves as a precursor to many of the other hormones, so even a slight deficiency can have a domino effect on other hormones.

CHAPTER 16:

Fasting for Hormone Balance

F asting, or more simply put, not eating, has been a healing practice for thousands of years. Over the last hundred years, our time between meals has gotten closer and closer together. It's gotten to the point where many people eat late at night and then eat breakfast first thing when they wake up in the morning. This isn't how our bodies were designed to eat, and it's not what will promote optimal functioning.

According to studies, it is likely that many of our genes were selected during the late Paleolithic era (50,000 to 10,000 B.C.), during a time when humans existed as hunter-gatherers. At that time there were no guarantees of finding food, resulting in mixed periods of feast and famine. This was just a fact of life. When there was food, we ate; when there was none, we fasted.

With that in mind, it makes sense that taking a break from eating is good for our hormones, our digestion, our brains and more. Currently, we are dealing with many diseases prompted by hormonal disruption such as diabetes, cardiac disease, autoimmune diseases, obesity, and even cancer. Fasting seems to be a promising tool in preventing and treating disease.

What is intermittent fasting?

Intermittent fasting simply means taking a break between meals. This break can be similar to a normal evening spent not eating (not eating from 7 p.m. to 7 a.m. would be a 12-hour fast), slightly longer (7 p.m. to 11 a.m. is a 16-hour fast), a 24-hour fast (not eating from dinner to dinner) or even several days. The type of fasting you practice depends on your individual body and preferences, in addition to what you're trying to accomplish. Many people prefer to simply skip breakfast, stretching out the period between dinner and their next meal, while others prefer the more extreme multi-day fasts, along with the spiritual and physiological benefits that come with it.

What hormones are affected by intermittent fasting?

Insulin

Insulin seems to respond extremely well to intermittent fasting. Although many of the initial studies on the benefits of fasting were done on animals, a recent human study showed improvement in insulin sensitivity. When you eat glucose and insulin levels spike, it triggers a number of actions in your body, such as helping cells in the liver, skeletal muscles, and fat tissue to absorb glucose from the blood. Once that is fulfilled, insulin signals the liver to take up glucose and store it as glycogen (stored energy) and then fat. If you keep spiking that insulin, you can get insulin resistance (cells get less sensitive to insulin) and in turn get inflammation, increased fat storage. By giving your body a "break" from the spikes, intermittent fasting allows the body to have better insulin sensitivity when you do eat, which in turn decreases inflammation, cortisol, excess estrogen and body fat.

Growth hormone (HGH)

Another hormone that is dramatically improved with fasting is human growth hormone (HGH), aka, the "Fountain of Youth" hormone. Growth hormones help preserve muscles and bone density and help us use fats for fuel. It also makes us look and feel "youthful" (depletion of HGH leads to wrinkles, saggy skin, gray and thinning hair, muscle loss, brain fog and low libido). Some athletes use it (illegally) for muscle growth and athletic performance. Unfortunately, natural growth hormone secretion decreases steadily as we age. One of the most potent stimuli to growth hormone secretion is fasting. Over a five-day fasting period, growth hormone secretion more than doubles.

Refer to the previous chapter on Human Growth Hormone to learn more about this youth giving hormone and how to boost it.

How to avoid feeling hungry and making your hormone imbalance worse

Intermittent fasting is extremely powerful for women who are over 35, in Perimenopause, Menopause or are dealing with insulin resistance, Auto-immunity or PCOS. However, if you're a woman on the thinner side, you need to be careful not to throw your hormones out of whack. Put simply, women are extremely sensitive to signals of external starvation. If the body senses that it is being starved, it will ramp up production of the hunger hormones leptin and ghrelin. When women experience insatiable hunger after undereating, they are actually experiencing the increased production of these hormones. It's the female body's way of protecting a potential fetus - even when a woman is not pregnant.

Prolonged, repeated, extended fasting can have negative effects on fertility and female hormones. In animal studies, after two weeks of intermittent fasting, female rats stopped having menstrual cycles and

their ovaries shrank, while they also experienced more insomnia than their male counterparts (though the male rats did experience lower testosterone production). The take-away? For everyone - but especially women - it's best to go low and slow. Start with a 12-hour fast two days a week, and if that feels comfortable, work your way up from there, adding an hour at a time. Listen to your body and remember, stress undoes any positive effects, so do only what's absolutely comfortable.

CHAPTER 17:

Detox for Hormone Balance

Most women I encounter have never thought about detoxification as related to their hormones. Most people are aware of detoxification (there are numerous detox protocols out there) and its benefits. However, most detoxes tend to focus on detoxification of the colon. There is nothing wrong with that, as a little colon detox from time to time can certainly come with its own benefits. But detoxification is about so much more.

Go into any health store and you will find a whole aisle of products aimed to cleanse or detoxify your liver, bowels and kidneys. But true detox requires more than popping a pill and sitting on the toilet.

So, what is a real detox?

Every single cell in your body has built-in detoxification methods. Your cells have the ability to take in the nutrients and the proteins and the chemicals from your bloodstream that they need for their particular function, and then release them back into circulation as waste products.

As I've mentioned before, our bodies are perfectly designed with all of the tools, equipment and innate intelligence to live happily on this planet. We were born with a built-in cleansing and waste removal system that allows our body to filter out and remove toxic substances taken in from our environment, as well as the bi-products of cellular metabolism. The liver, kidneys, intestines, skin and lymphatic system are major players in the body's detoxification system and they are constantly working to filter toxins that can be excreted through sweat, breath, urine and stool.

With these systems in place, some may view cleansing and detox practices as "fads" or unnecessary treatments, because our organs are made to filter themselves all of the time. However, in this day and age, we are constantly taking in toxins and other nasty stuff that our bodies are not used to dealing with. For example, the processed foods, plastics, unnatural body care products, scented candles, mercury fillings, chemical laden cleaning products, flame retardants, fluoridated water, and pollution we encounter is new to us as a species, especially in the amounts we are exposed to today.

Our bodies are simply not designed to filter these types of toxins and in these quantities. When toxins accumulate, it is bad news for us and our hormones.

Here are just a few ways that toxicity can affect your hormones:

- Toxic buildup increases inflammation and cortisol levels. This affects blood sugar and lowers the production of estrogen and progesterone.
- Reducing toxic load improves hormone creation and filtration
- Decreasing body fat stabilizes hormones
- Reducing toxic load reduces inflammation and decreases cortisol levels

As far as toxic buildup increasing cortisol levels, we all know that cortisol is the "stress" hormone, and that too much can cause dreaded "belly fat" to accumulate around our mid-section. Extra fat in this area is a major risk factor for diabetes, cardiovascular disease, estrogen dominance and infertility, to name a few. Extra weight in this area is also particularly hard to get rid of. When we are chronically stressed, cortisol levels get out of whack.

Excess cortisol also causes tons of inflammation to build up in our bodies. This causes excess glucose to build up in our blood, increasing the amount of hunger, mood swings, and energy dips we experience. This can lead to insulin resistance, PCOS, Diabetes and obesity. With our body constantly battling to reduce this inflammation, hormone production falls to the wayside and our body's ability to make estrogen, progesterone and testosterone is impaired.

112

In addition to removing toxins and chemicals from your food and environment, you will also want to work on eliminating toxic thoughts, toxic relationships, and incorporating some of the movement patterns, breathing exercises, and implementing some of the toxin reduction tips and tools found in the 21 Days to Hormone Harmony plan following this chapter.

The key is to be kind and gentle to your body and to incorporate practices into your daily routine that promote detoxification.

Eating plenty of plant-based alkaline foods and decreasing potentially allergenic foods such as gluten, dairy and soy for a period of time allows your body to rebuild. When this happens, we are better able to make and filter the right types and amounts of hormones.

A major part of being healthy is to ensure that any toxins that enter our system are effectively identified by the body and escorted out in a harmless fashion. There are many systems, organs, and glands in place to make sure this occurs, but unfortunately, many of them have become clogged and compromised to the point of complete dysfunction. One of those important systems that aid in the removal of toxins and has become clogged in many ways, is the lymphatic system.

The lymphatic system is a complex drainage or system. You can think of it as a "sewer system" that consists of glands, lymph nodes, the spleen, thymus gland, and tonsils. Its role is to cleanse our cells by absorbing excess fluids, fats, and toxins from our tissues and into the blood where it can eventually be filtered out by the liver and kidneys.

Unfortunately, due to our increased toxic burden, nutritional deficiencies and sedentary lifestyles, this system has become increasingly polluted. If you suffer from any of the following, it may be a sign that your lymphatic system is clogged and needs a serious cleanse:

- Skin conditions
- Arthritis
- Unexplained injuries
- Excess weight or cellulite
- Headaches

- Chronic fatigue

- Sinus infections

- Digestive disorders

- Enlarged lymph nodes

If you identify with any of these conditions, you will want to strongly consider incorporating the following 10 factors to help detoxify your lymphatic system.

Exercise

If you have a toxic lymphatic system, the best approach is to start slow on the exercise and be consistent. One of the easiest, safest, and most profound exercises you can incorporate is rebounding. This is the simple act of lightly bouncing up and down on a "mini trampoline", which is the perfect movement for stimulating lymph flow, and toning other detoxification organs as well. You can learn more about rebounding in the 21 Days to Hormone Harmony section at the end of this book.

Sauna

An infrared sauna is also an excellent and easy option, as the sweat excreted through your skin can help release the toxic burden on your lymphatic system and allow it to work more effectively.

Hot and cold showers

Although it may not sound like fun, a hot and cold shower can be effective when it comes to benefiting the lymphatic system. The hot water helps dilate the blood vessels, and the cold contracts them, creating a "pump" action that helps force fluid that may be stagnant in the system.

Since your lymph system has no central pump of its own, this therapy -and others which stimulate this type of action- are great solutions to get it flowing properly again. Caution is required when using this therapy if you have a heart condition or are pregnant.

Dry brushing

Using a natural bristle brush, brush your dry skin in a circular motion before showering. Start with your feet and move towards the torso and do the same from your fingers to the chest. You want to flow in the same direction as your lymph circulates, towards the heart.

This stimulates the lymphatic system into action and helps open up the pores for easier toxin removal. A hot and cold shower after this dry brushing session would be ideal.

Drink adequate amounts of clean pure water

You've heard it before: Drink your water! However, I must point out that if you don't properly source your water, you're actively adding to your toxic burden by ingesting easily absorbed toxins often present in water such as fluoride, chlorine, VOC's, and more.

So, ensure you are investing in a filtration system proven to work well or look to get spring water from an approved source free of these types of contaminants. Go to Findaspring.com for a source near you. Then you can safely consume up to a gallon of water a day, with minimum consumption at just ½ your body weight in ounces (Example, if you weigh 150 lbs., you would drink a minimum of 75 ounces).

Avoid restrictive clothing

It's important not to wear tight clothing that can cut off proper circulation within the lymphatic system. This can cause blockages to occur and toxins to build up in different areas of the body.

Areas of particular importance where this may occur is bras for women that may be too tight in the axillary lymph node area (armpit area), and in the inguinal lymph node area (groin) where tight fitting underwear could cause a problem over time. Bras with underwires are especially problematic due to their constriction of lymphatic flow.

Now, I don't want to cramp your style, and if you already have a killer outfit picked out for a special occasion, you can go for it. It's fine to wear something tight from time to time, but avoid being excessive and keep the bra off as much as possible. If you must wear one, consider a bra that doesn't contain an underwire to improve the flow dramatically.

Breathe deeply

Another method of "pumping" lymph properly comes from deep breathing. Since our bodies have 3x more lymph fluid than blood, this exercise becomes increasingly important in order to get the toxins into the blood and be detoxified by your liver and kidneys.

So breathe deeply from your belly and exhale smoothly to facilitate this process. I'll show you exactly how to do this later in this book.

Eat foods that promote lymph flow

Eating a clean, nutrient rich diet rooted in produce is the first step to promoting healthy lymph flow. Some particularly cleansing foods for the lymphatic system include:

- Dark leafy greens
- Low sugar fruits
- Garlic
- Ground flaxseed
- Seaweed
- Algae
- Chia
- Avocados
- Cranberries
- Walnuts
- Brazil nuts
- Almonds

These types of foods will help provide the necessary vitamins, minerals, EFA's, and enzymes to cleanse your lymphatic system more efficiently.

Also, avoid foods, personal care products, and environments that cause lymph stagnation. This means avoiding conventional personal care products loaded with parabens, petroleum, and phthalates, and staying out of heavily polluted areas by opting for more oxygen rich environments.

In addition to that, avoiding the following foods are critical to improving your lymphatic health:

- Sugar
- Artificial sweeteners
- Conventional dairy
- Conventionally raised meat
- Refined grains
- Processed foods
- Soy
- Preservatives and additives
- Table salt
- Baked goods

As with most chronic conditions, a multi-faceted lifestyle approach is often the only way to do a proper clean-up of any system, and that goes for the lymphatic system as well. So, be sure to layer in all of these factors for a much more comprehensive cleanse and enjoy the improved health that comes with rejuvenating a clogged lymphatic system.

The Liver

"Happy Liver, Happy Life" – an adage from Chinese Medicine

The liver is the largest internal organ. Do you know where it is found? Put your right hand over the end of your right rib cage, just below the diaphragm – your hand is now over your liver.

Your liver performs about 200 vital functions, most of which are vital for good health. This includes the conversion of hormones, as well as detoxification of the blood, protein synthesis, excretion of bilirubin, cholesterol, drugs, and production of bile (an alkaline compound which helps in digestion through the emulsification of lipids), which are just some of the important functions that the liver performs.

This means that reducing Toxic Load Improves Hormone Creation and Filtration.

Our livers are so wonderful. They store, create and filter so many different substances in our bodies. When we encounter and consume a lot of toxins over time, such as processed foods, unnatural body care products, or smog from the air, our livers get overloaded. When they are stuffed full of nonsense, they can't do their job effectively. What does this mean to you?

It means imbalanced hormones! Which means our periods are irregular, we seem to age faster, mood swings and hot flashes become the norm and we wake up every night around 3 am and have trouble getting back to sleep.

The liver synthesizes and secretes at least four important hormones (which you may not have heard of). They are:

- Insulin-like Growth Factor-1 (IGF-1) – necessary for growth and cellular repair

- Angiotensinogen – plays a role in maintaining blood pressure

- Thrombopoietin - plays a role in the generation of platelets, essential for blood clotting

- Hepcidin – Helps to maintain homeostatic levels of iron in your body fluids and is part of the body's innate immune system, acting as a defense against pathogens

- Betatrophin – stimulates the proliferation of the insulin producing beta cells in the pancreas - vital for blood sugar balance

The Liver also breaks down the steroid hormones which include:

- The sex hormones: estrogen, progesterone, and testosterone, which control our body shape, energy, and sex life to name a few things
- Aldosterone, which controls the balance of the mineral's sodium and potassium along with fluid balance
- Cortisone, which plays large role in immune health, among many other functions

The liver is also responsible for the production of 60% of your active thyroid hormone. The thyroid itself only produces 7% of the body's active hormone. The Inactive thyroid hormone (T4) is converted into the active form T3 in the liver by process of conjugation.

Phase I and Phase II Pathways

The liver metabolizes hormones and other substances using two primary phases known as the Phase I and Phase II pathways.

During Phase I, some hormones or substances are metabolized directly, but others are converted into intermediate forms, which are then further metabolized in Phase II.

These two phases of biological transformation are how the liver provides the body with nutrients and supports the excretion of excess or toxic substances through the urine, liver bile, perspiration and exhaled air.

In the example of estrogen, the Phase I pathway is the main metabolic pathway for the estrogen hormones. In pre-menopausal women, the ovaries produce estrogen, primarily estradiol, most of which the body converts to estrone, and eventually estriol. The liver then metabolizes the remaining estradiol and the converted estrone, breaking it down further, and excreting the excess from the body.

Some researchers and practitioners now believe that the liver's ability to metabolize estrone is the key to understanding estrogen-related cancer risk.

During Phase I metabolism, estrone is converted into various metabolites including 2-hydroxyestrone, a very weak estrogen, and 16-alphahydroxyestrone, a very potent estrogen. If the conversion process favors the stronger form(s) rather than the weaker form(s), then tissue that has an abundance of estrogen receptors, such as the breasts and uterus, may be more vulnerable to excessive estrogen activity, potentially leading to the formation of fibroids or the stimulation of estrogen-sensitive cancers.

Phase I processing can be affected by many factors, including extreme toxic overload, the effects of alcohol or drugs, a lack of nutrients, genetic variation, or interference from other substances.

Many prescription drugs are metabolized in Phase I, which can also interfere with the liver's ability to handle the estrogen hormones. On the other hand, DIM, also known as, Indole-3-carbinol (I3C), a phytonutrient derived from cruciferous vegetables (e.g., broccoli, cauliflower, cabbage and Brussels sprouts), stimulates enzymes that promote the metabolism of estrogens into milder forms, potentially reducing the risk of estrogen-dependent cancers.

During Phase II, a process known as conjugation begins in which nutrients such as amino acids are combined with hormones and other substances to convert them into water-soluble compounds that can be excreted efficiently in the urine or stool.

Of the various types of conjugation that may occur in Phase II, the following are most relevant to hormone metabolism:

Methylation, also known as methyl metabolism, is the process in which small parts of molecules, called methyl groups, are passed from one molecule to another. Once estrogens are methylated, they can be easily excreted. In order for the liver to have an adequate supply of methyl groups available, an adequate intake of vitamins B6 (e.g., nuts, veggies, liver) and B12 (primarily from animal products), and folate (such as from green leafy vegetables) are necessary. An over-the-counter dietary supplement known as Mors is a methyl donor, supplying methyl groups.

Sulfation is the process in which sulfur groups are added to estrogen or other molecules to prepare them for easy excretion. Adequate amounts of foods containing sulfur should be in the diet, including egg yolks, garlic, onions and Brussels sprouts. Animal protein is another important source of sulfur.

Free Radicals

Each reaction in the Phase I pathway produces an intermediate form called a free radical. As you have probably heard, free radicals can be very damaging to body tissues if they are not quickly neutralized by antioxidants. Nutrients such as Vitamins C and E, minerals such as selenium, and other substances such as NAC, lipoic acid and glutathione are antioxidants that help protect against free radicals. The intermediate forms produced in Phase I are in a highly reactive state until they are fully converted in Phase II.

Glucuronidation is another process by which estrogens can be conjugated. This type of conjugation may be affected by the condition of the intestines. If the intestines have an abundance of abnormal bacteria, an enzyme produced by these bacteria may cut off the conjugated part from the estrogen. The estrogen that would have been excreted is then reabsorbed back into the body, allowing even estrogens produced by the body to build up to excessive levels. The supplement calcium d-glucarate (also found in fruits and vegetables) can render the enzyme inactive and prevent this build-up.

Glutathione conjugation is the process in which glutathione, another sulfur-containing molecule, is added to estrogen for easy excretion. Foods such as avocado, walnuts and asparagus are rich in glutathione, and vitamin C stimulates the body to produce more of it. Glutathione depletion can be due to a lack of the essential nutrients and amino acids (found in fresh fruits, vegetables, fish and meats) that are needed to synthesize it.

Glutathione deserves special mention as a crucial detoxifier because it also behaves as an antioxidant in Phase I. Glutathione neutralizes the free radicals produced in the Phase I reactions and combines with them to produce water-soluble compounds that can be excreted.

121

Glutathione is also needed for the detoxification of alcohol. Studies have shown that even a small amount of alcohol intake can increase estrogen levels in the blood because alcohol competes for the available glutathione, preventing estrogen excretion.

Smoking is also known to deplete glutathione levels, as do chronically stressful conditions such as infections or inflammatory disorders.

It is important to note that excess toxins that the liver cannot conjugate are stored in the fat, where they are locked away.

A simple genetic panel can give you a great deal of insight into your body's ability to metabolize hormones effectively and guide protocols the enhance detoxification.

Decreasing Body Fat Increases Energy and Stabilizes Hormones

When you do a cleanse, you are dumping waste that has accumulated in your body. Often, this leads to accelerated weight loss and easier weight management. When we reduce our body fat into healthy ranges, the toxins we encounter in our daily lives have less room to be stored. No toxin storage room equals better health, increased energy and a whole host of other amazing benefits.

When you have more energy, you are more likely to stick with the healthy lifestyle choices that make you feel great. Your hormones are more likely to be made on time and in the right amounts. Excesses are less likely be stored which means a sizable reduction in hot flashes, period cramps, irritability, brain fog, weight gain or other nasty symptoms you experience right now.

Now, I wouldn't tell you all of this and then leave you to your own devices. The purpose of this book is not only to inspire a transformation, but also to help you achieve one.

Now that you have a working knowledge of hormones, what they are, what they do, how they change and the type of things we can do to keep them balanced, I invite you to join me in the remaining section of this book in my *21 Days to Hormone Harmony* protocol. You'll find everythingyou need to support healthy detoxification and hormone balance; from recipes to meal plans to kitchen prep tips, to at-home treatments. This is a great place to start and to give your hormones and body a much-needed detox and jump-start.

Be sure to take the Hormone Harmony Assessment, found in Section 1, before and after completing the 21-day program, and again 4 weeks later.

About Dr. Michelle Sands

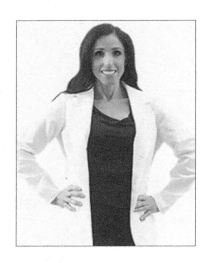

D r. Michelle Sands is a #1 International Best-Selling Author, licensed Functional Medicine Physician, Doctor of Naturopathic Medicine (ND) and highly sought-after Female Hormone and Epigenetics Expert. Dr. Michelle, her book and programs, have been featured on ABC, CBS, Outside Magazine, The Boston Herald, NBC, Fox News and USA Today. She is the founder and co-owner of Glow Natural Wellness and creator of The Glow Protocol. But, first and foremost, she is a loving wife and a proud mom.

It wasn't long ago that she struggled with autoimmunity, digestive issues, chronic pain, acne, and anxiety. Diagnosed with Primary Ovarian Failure at the age of 20, her doctor explained that she would never have children of her own. Michelle was devastated. She was given a handful of prescriptions, but zero solutions. After decades of research, trial and error, medical school, interning, testing, and prayer, she was finally able to understand what her body was trying to tell her. She shifted her focus from symptoms to systems and began to heal. On April 5th, 2015, she gave birth to her miracle baby, Paxton Emerson Sands, naturally.

Dr. Michelle believes that nature provides us with everything we need to heal our bodies and live optimally. She also understands that in today's modern world our bodies and minds are exposed to lots of unnatural things that take away from that optimal level of health.

Dr. Sands is passionate about helping women to harness the power of nature and leverage their unique genetics, so they can live vibrantly, not just optimizing health physically, but mentally, emotionally and spiritually as well. Her goal for all women is for them to love their bodies and enjoy their lives. GLOW stands for Genetic Leveraging For Optimal Wellness and Dr. Sands uses modern science, functional lab testing, holistic lifestyle medicine, natural supplementation, epigenetic coaching, and eastern philosophies to restore health and increase vital energy in every woman she works with.

Today, Dr. Sands sees women from all over the world in her virtual practice, Glow Natural Wellness, and has a remarkable track record for improving health and happiness with her proprietary system, The Glow Protocol.

Dr. Michelle enjoys an active lifestyle and is a 7-time Ironman triathlon finisher, ultra-marathoner, former competitive kickboxer, world champion adventure racer and an active, fun-loving mom.

Work with Dr. Michelle

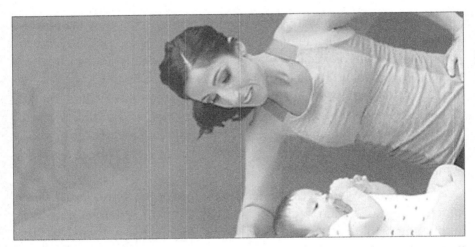

Balance Your Hormones, Leverage Your Genetics and Reach Your Full Potential with Dr. Michelle's most popular program The GLOW Protocol

Help is here. What you need is a customized plan, the right tools and support from a knowledgeable medical professional who understands what you're going through.

Take control of your health simply and effectively by following my proven 5-step system called The GLOW Protocol. Perhaps you've seen some of the media coverage documenting the extraordinary results achieved in this program by women just like you.

To ensure a smooth transformation, you'll gain access to cutting edge functional medicine tools, state of the art laboratory testing and the support of North America's top female functional medicine expert.

I will help you build a strong foundation, understand the root cause of your symptoms, and then guide you through my proven healing protocols so you can HEAL, GROW and THRIVE.

https://glownaturalwellness.com/glow

Resources

Online Dispensary - FullScript - create a free account to gain access to discounted pharmaceutical grade supplements, and Dr. Michelle's top picks. https://us.fullscript.com//welcome/msands

Epigenetic Testing and Coaching - streamline and fast track your results with precise and strategic supplement, nutrition, activity and lifestyle plans based on your unique genetic code and your personal goals. Watch my Masterclass: https://glownaturalwellness.com/joindnamadesimple

Consumer Direct Blood Testing - Don't wait for you doc to order tests for you. Get answers now. Order your own test and get your own result that you can take to any doctor. Contact us at support@glownaturalwellness.com

Section III

21 Days to Hormone Harmony (AKA The 21 Day Metabolic Rehab and Hormone Makeover)

The pages that follow contain all the materials, information, guidelines, recipes, meal plans, shopping lists, daily protocol sheets, supplements, exercise, detoxification and stress reduction recommendations that you need to successfully complete this hormone detox and metabolic recovery program.

I've included a guidebook, so you know what to do, when to do it and why. You'll also find a workbook to help you document your progress.

If you need additional support, please join my private community, The GLOW Tribe, where you can ask questions. Or, if you are a visual and auditory learner, you can purchase the digital course here. The digital program gives you lifetime access to our members' portal where you will find video tutorials, downloadable worksheets and handouts as well as bonus materials to support you on your journey. As an added bonus, those who purchase the digital program will also get a complimentary 30-minute wrap up call with Dr. Michelle or a member of her team.

Remember, everything you need to successfully complete the 3-week program is in the pages that follow. And it is not necessary to purchase the digital program. Only do so if you know you need additional support.

Let's dive in! You will find the following materials on this final section of this book:

21 Days to Hormone Harmony Guide Book

Meal Plans and Recipe Guides

Shopping Lists

Daily Protocol Sheets

Toxin Reduction Tools

Kitchen and Meal Prep Tips

Metabolic Meditations

Will You Leave a Book Review?

Did you enjoy this book and find it useful?
I will be very grateful when you post a short review and give your success story on Amazon right now!

Your support makes a difference. I *read and respond to all the reviews personally* to make this book even better!

To leave a review right now, go here:
http://bit.ly/reviewHH35

21 Days to Hormone Harmony Guidebook

This guidebook is designed to give you the basic knowledge upon which to build a strong foundation for your health and achieve a natural state of radiance, energy, and balance. You will be able to use this guidebook again and again as you deepen your understanding of your own needs for metabolic healing, detoxification and optimum wellness.

Even those who have a super clean diet and lifestyle benefit from a seasonal rehab or detox because of modern day stressors and toxins we cannot always control. No matter your current lifestyle, health level, diet, or energy level, regular detoxification can be a very special gift to give to yourself.

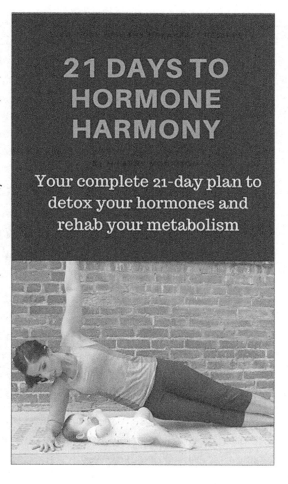

21 DAYS TO HORMONE HARMONY

Your complete 21-day plan to detox your hormones and rehab your metabolism

Many of us set aside time to spring clean our homes, our yards, and our automobiles. Yet the body is often forgotten. This is a wonderful opportunity to support your body so it may function at its full potential. I see many patients who suffer from allergies, stress, fatigue, headaches, hormonal imbalances, digestive issues, weak immune systems, weight loss resistance and skin problems. These symptoms are your body crying for help. It is asking for a time to rest, rejuvenate, be deeply nurtured and "rehabilitated." During this program, you will need to invest a little extra time and attention into self-care, but your reward will be feeling like you have a new lease on life.

> *Disclaimer: The contents of this booklet are based on the knowledge, opinions, and experience of Dr. Michelle Sands, ND, unless otherwise noted. The information in this handout does not replace a one-on-one relationship with a qualified health care professional and should not be considered medical advice. Dr. Michelle encourages you to make your own health care decisions based on your research and in partnership with a qualified health care professional. And most importantly, make sure to listen to your body.*

Why Should You Do a Hormone Detox or Rehab?

As we age, our metabolism begins to slow down. This is because the energy powerhouses in our cells, known as mitochondria, begin to disappear. A slower metabolism means less energy and more fat gain, even if you are eating the same foods you always do.

Part of the rehab is detoxification. Imagine if you lived in a very small space, what would it be like if you could only remove 20% of the trash you brought in? What would it feel like to be in that space after a week? What about a month? Now imagine a year! How does it feel to be in that space now? This is how your cells feel when they cannot release waste.

Detoxing your cells will improve your ability to absorb nutrients and eliminate waste. It will also stabilize and improve your energy. During this program, you will improve your health, increase your energy, and eliminate waste that causes disease, weight gain, and cravings.

When your body cannot eliminate waste properly, it becomes acidic and toxic. When it becomes acidic and toxic, your blood and your cells slow down and those mitochondria can't do their jobs. When this happens, your body starts to slow down, you gain weight and become more susceptible to illness and chronic disease.

There are three reasons why toxins build up in your body.

- You take in more than you can eliminate either with food or life-style, which inhibits your body from being able to fully recover
- Toxins in your food, your environment, and your thoughts create waste your body cannot use
- An overly acidic diet allows micro-organisms (yeasts, molds, fun-guses, etc.) and produces Mycotoxins in your body, which makes more toxins

Toxins are stored in your cells and the quality of your life comes down to the quality of your cells.

Healthy Cells: Because cells are vital to all life, they have basic needs for their survival. Essentially, there are four things cells need, not just to survive, but to thrive:

- Oxygen
- Water – the most abundant substance in the body
- Nutrition (chemical information that tells the cells how to behave)
- The ability to eliminate waste

Your blood transports oxygen and nutrients to your tissues and eliminates waste. Your lymph system works closely with the circulatory system as it cleanses and returns tissue fluid to the blood and destroys toxins that enter your body. Your body has three times more lymph fluid than blood.

This program is designed to help you improve the quality of your cells and the mitochondria within them by improving how your cells receive oxygen, water, and nutrients, and how your cells eliminate waste.

Toxins and Inflammation

To achieve health, radiance, energy, balance, and permanent weight loss, it is helpful to understand the underlying causes of diseases and obesity, which are toxins and inflammation. The good news is that we can restrict these causes by choosing to take an active role in feeling and looking better. A great way to do this is with metabolic cleansing and rebuilding. Ninety percent of the time, I start my clients on a metabolic rehab, because it brings balance to your body and improves your digestive system, enabling you to be more successful with future health goals. But before we begin our Metabolic Rehab, let's talk a little bit about toxins and inflammation.

What makes us toxic?

Certain foods, our environment, and even our lifestyle make us toxic. The simple truth is, we are surrounded by toxins. In fact, we are exposed to more environmental toxins in one day than our grandparents were in an entire lifetime. Environmental chemicals in solvents, plastics, and adhesives; poisons in makeup, moisturizers, nail polish, hair dyes, and shampoos; pesticides, herbicides, parasites in soil, food, and water; ingestible chemicals in junk and processed foods; the toxins released by our bodies when under consistent stress; and even the toxic thoughts and words we may subject ourselves to on a daily basis all contribute to an ever-increasing lack of radiance and energy.

What creates inflammation?

Sugar, lack of exercise, toxins, food allergies, and food sensitivities all cause inflammation. Inflammation causes weight gain and prevents weight loss. It's a vicious cycle – being inflamed makes you fat and being fat makes you inflamed.

Problems that can result from toxic overload and inflammation:

- Bad breath
- Bloating, gas, constipation, and diarrhea
- Canker sores
- Difficulty concentrating
- Excess weight or difficulty losing weight
- Fatigue
- Fluid retention
- Food cravings
- Headaches
- Heartburn
- Joint pain
- Muscle aches
- Puffy eyes and dark circles
- Postnasal drip
- Sinus congestion
- Skin rashes and acne
- Sleep problems
- Toxins can also block thyroid function, impair female hormones, and may account for depression, anxiety, and fatigue

The results you should experience in this program:

- Weight loss
- More energy
- Better digestion and elimination
- Fewer symptoms of chronic illness

- Improved concentration and mental clarity
- Less congestion and fewer allergy-related systems
- Less joint pain
- Less fluid retention
- Increased sense of peace and relaxation
- Enhanced sleep
- Better looking skin
- Brighter eyes
- Clearer Mind and ability to focus
- An overall sense of well-being

<u>Let's Get Started!</u>

Preparation

Complete the "Before You Begin" section of your Workbook BEFORE moving on (link to download the guidebook is below).

Get organized. Read the program materials provided and input new habits, self-care, and routines into your calendar. Try to automate everything as much as possible.

Go shopping for the food supplies described in the program.

Create a system to make things easy. Set up your needed utensils, wash and cut vegetables, etc. Put away all items you will not need to create a cleanse-friendly environment. Set aside time to complete your workbook and get in touch with your goals.

Benefits of this Hormone Detox and Metabolic Rehab

There are many reasons a person may choose to reboot their metabolism. As you go through this process, you will find that even if you started off with just one reason, the benefits you experience are often broader and further-reaching.

Cleansing or detoxifying alone, however, is not the solution. Getting rid of the toxins and minimizing exposure to new toxins must always be balanced with replenishing the body's vitamin, mineral, and macronutrient reserves. When we simply cleanse without rebuilding, it is like removing the old oil from your car without replenishing it with new oil. Your body will be running on empty.

In addition to nutrition, we must concentrate on cleansing and rebuilding the mind, our relationship with food, and our bodies.

Summary of potential benefits:

- Increased energy
- Mental clarity
- Improved digestion
- Allergy relief
- Weight loss
- Hormonal balance
- Radiant skin
- Improved physical appearance
- Longevity and disease prevention
- Relief from minor health conditions
- Clarity in life path and goals
- Tissue regeneration
- Increased general wellbeing
- Personal confidence and empowerment

This is a gentle and relatively short program designed to jump-start your journey to health. The diet may seem fairly restrictive compared to the modern-day American diet, but you should not go hungry as this is not a fast. Eat abundantly from the foods that are listed for each phase of the program and use the menus and recipes as guides to make the most of your experience.

139

**You do not have to use every recipe or eat every food on the list. Most people find a few "go to" recipes for breakfast, lunch and dinner. However, I have provided you with plenty of options – so you don't get bored or feel deprived.

This program is designed to be gentle, yet effective. It is also intended to be doable while you work, play, take care of your family or go about your normal day. Your normal routine, however, will be a bit different during this program, simply because you will be eating, doing and thinking different things while rehabilitating your metabolism.

One incredible benefit will be the awareness gained about how different foods make you feel physically, emotionally, and energetically. Your taste buds will begin to change, and you will begin to understand how your body is responding to the foods you are consuming. This will give you more control of reactions you were not aware were caused by foods.

There are thousands of different dietary recommendations and philosophies, and new ones come up every day. The very best way to figure out your personalized diet is to begin to pay attention to how you feel as you explore different ways of eating and being. In the process of the program, you will begin to recognize which foods may not be serving you, despite what you have read or been told. With that said, this program is based on whole, real foods.

Cleansing and your body

Every toxin you come into contact with must be filtered through the liver. The liver is the second largest organ in your body and it is also the most overworked. Given that we now understand the degree to which we are exposed to toxins on a daily basis, it is easy to see how our livers are being put into overdrive. When the liver becomes overburdened, it loses its ability to function efficiently. This leads to a cascade of potentially serious health consequences and uncomfortable reactions.

What happens when the liver is not functioning properly or is overburdened? Toxins begin to find their way into other organs, skin, fatty tissues, and the blood. This is when we begin to see and feel the manifestation of some of the common ailments described above.

The detoxification strategies we will implement are focused on cleansing the liver. However, they will also provide support to other systems in your body, such as the colon, skin, lymph, lungs, kidneys and bladder, mind and emotions. As the liver starts the process to release toxins, these other organ systems will also provide pathways to efficient elimination. In Phase 2 of the program, you will drink a special simple olive oil and lemon juice cocktail to promote liver detoxification by increasing bile flow first thing every morning.

Common Signs That the Liver May Need Some Attention

Do you wake up at night?

If you wake up consistently between 1:00am and 3:00am, your liver may be asking for some support. While we sleep, the liver becomes more active and works on cleansing and detoxification. Waking up around this "liver time" can signal that the liver is exhibiting signs of toxicity and needs some cleansing. Many times, this happens from eating either too much sugar in the evening or animal protein.

Eye problems?

Conjunctivitis, lots of mucus, itching, macular degeneration, dry eyes, and cataracts indicate liver weakness. Another physical clue is a vertical line between the eyebrows.

Skin problems?

Eczema, psoriasis, rosacea, skin rashes, acne and dry skin are clues.

Angry emotions?

If the liver is congested and being forced to work too hard, it becomes "hot," causing excessive anger and irritation.

Hormonal imbalances?

PMS, hot flashes, and pre-menopausal symptoms are increased due to a congested liver.

Constipation?

This condition can often be caused by a congested and toxic liver or even stressed adrenals. The colon should still be addressed, but it is often not the root cause.

10 Steps that Support a Healthy Liver

- Eliminate toxins from your diet and your life as best you can

- Drink pure (filtered) water throughout the day

- Drink your lemon water first thing every morning

- Eat dark greens, preferably raw, every day (e.g. "green juice," a big or a green salad). Eat lots of celery (a good source of plant sodium that helps support the adrenals), watercress, broccoli, kale, cucumber, spinach, romaine, fresh herbs like basil and cilantro, and sour green apples.

- Eat animal protein between 10 a.m. and 3 p.m. It can be stressful for the liver to eat the animal protein later in the day or evening, especially if you are showing signs of liver stress. Everyone is different, and some people may have no problem cleansing animal protein later in the day. If you are unsure, stick with the guidelines we lay out for you.

- Remember, you need protein to support and detoxify the liver. In addition to protein naturally found in foods, good complete protein sources can be found in beans, nuts, and seeds such as hemp seeds and chia seeds (I can hear the paleo police writing my ticket right now- but I do feel that beans can be a great – and inexpensive - protein source when prepared properly).

- Eat dinner at least 2-3 hours before bedtime

- Make sure the colon is supported and clean. When toxins remain in the colon, they are sent back to the liver. The liver then sends them right back down to the colon in the bile. To help permanently eliminate these toxins from the body, add extra fiber, probiotics, and filtered water.

- Sweat! Saunas and exercise are a good way to sweat. Another way is the toxin elimination bath (details provided in your resources) at least 3-4 times per week.

- Assist your lymphatic system - Use a body brush every day to stimulate your lymphatic system and help move lymphatic fluids. You can also jump on a mini trampoline, which is a way to stimulate lymphatic drainage, ridding your body of toxins, wastes, trapped protein, bacteria, and viruses. Another name for this is rebounding. This creates an ideal condition for cleaning the cells. The vertical acceleration and deceleration help the cells squeeze out waste.

Your Hormone Detox

I have outlined the basic program below. If you have any specific issues, such as inflammation, candida, cellulite, hormonal issues, possible food intolerances, allergies, or blood sugar issues such as hypoglycemia and insulin resistance, I can provide you additional information to support these conditions. Please let me know and we can schedule a one-on-one session to discuss.

The three phases of this program:

Phase 1 – Mental and physical preparation, elimination of negative thoughts, refined foods and stimulants.

Phase 2 – Deepening the detox, stimulating metabolism, allowing for digestive repair and liver detox, elimination of troublesome foods. Optional 3-day lemonade fast.

Phase 3 – Adding and awareness.

How to optimize your Hormone Harmony Detox

- It is ideal to space meals 3-4 hours apart. This allows the body to tap into and begin to burn fatty tissue that is storing toxins.

- Eat your evening meal at least 2-3 hours before going to bed to ensure that you are not still digesting when your body needs its rest and renewal. The body, particularly the liver, does some serious detoxing at night. This is why staying up past midnight to party (alcohol, drugs) is particularly destructive to the liver.

Hormone Harmony Foods

On the program you will be eating only the foods on the "good food" list below, while including at least some of the suggested therapies and lifestyle habits.

Foods you will enjoy during most phases (If marked with ** avoid this food during Phase 2.).

- ** Fish, especially small, non-predatory species such as sardines, herring, wild salmon, cod (and black cod), and sole
- ** Lean white chicken (preferably organic)
- **Eggs (preferably pasture raised)
- Fresh or frozen non-citrus fruit, ideally berries (only organic)
- Fresh vegetables – no limit, try to eat more than four cups per day
- Legumes - lentils, navy beans, adzuki beans, mung beans, and others (please use organic and soak dry beans before preparing)
- Brown rice and quinoa (during Phase 2 limit to two servings daily)
- Unsalted raw nuts and seeds (no peanuts)
- Flaxseeds (ground)
- Lemons - organic, do not purchase pre-squeezed lemon juice
- Lemon and olive oil cocktail (1 tablespoon of organic extra virgin olive oil and half a squeezed lemon)
- Vegetable broth (organic and sugar-free)
- Sea vegetables

- Avocados
- Olive oil
- Coconut oil
- Raw apple cider vinegar
- Herbal teas
- Unsweetened cranberry juice

Foods and substances to avoid during all phases:

- Sugar (white sugar, cane sugar, dehydrated cane juice, brown sugar, honey, maple syrup, high fructose corn syrup, sucrose, glucose, maltose, dextrose, lactose, corn syrup, and white grape juice concentrate)

- Sugar alcohols such as sorbitol, mannitol, xylitol, and maltitol
- Artificial sweeteners like aspartame
- Natural sweeteners (Stevia is ok to include)
- Alcohol
- Caffeine (except green tea)
- Citrus fruits and juice (except lemon juice and unsweetened cranberry juice)
- Yeast (baker's and brewer's), fermented foods (including vinegar, except raw apple cider vinegar)
- Dairy products
- No fermented soy products (e.g. miso, tempeh – Gluten-free tamari is ok)
- Dried fruits (dates, prunes, raisins, figs, etc.)
- Gluten (anything made with wheat) and all flour products
- Corn
- Nightshade plants (tomatoes, potatoes, eggplants, bell peppers)

145

- Peanuts
- Refined oils and hydrogenated fats such as margarine
- Stimulants
- Processed foods or food additives
- Fast food
- Junk food
- Any food that comes in a box, package, or is commercially prepared

A note about probiotics:

Probiotics are included on your daily protocol because they are essential for optimal digestion of food and absorption of nutrients, and they help your body produce vitamins, absorb minerals and aid in the elimination of toxins. Not all probiotics are the same! My favorite is Megasporebiotic. You can order through Fullscript: https://us.fullscript.com//welcome/msands

All 3 Phases

Phase 1: Preparation (7 days)

To begin to prepare the body, you will eliminate sugar, dairy, refined foods, refined oils, and coffee. You will also want to prepare your environment and collect the foods, tools, supplies, and supplements you will need. As you go through this preparation, you will experience the strongest and most frequent signs of toxic withdrawal.

What is toxic withdrawal?

When you start to eliminate substances that your body has become dependent upon (addictive substances), your body will naturally respond and ask for them back. It doesn't do this in a comfortable or easy way. It is important for you to realize that only unhealthy, toxic substances are addictive. If you experience uncomfortable sensations, these are signals that repair is under way and the removal of toxins from your body is occurring.

146

The more you search for fast, temporary relief with a candy bar, soda, or chips, the more you will inhibit the healing detoxification process.

Signs you are experiencing toxic withdrawal are:

- Headache
- Weakness
- Stomach cramping
- Lightheadedness
- Empty, growling stomach
- Irritability, moodiness
- Fatigue
- Bloated feeling

Depending on your situation, these symptoms can last from two to five days. This will be the most difficult part of the program, but these changes are the most important in getting you started. Don't give up!

Phase 2: Deep Cellular Cleaning /Alkalizing the Body (7 days)

In this phase, avoid animal protein, restrict oil intake to no more than 2 tablespoons per day of coconut oil or flax oil (except for the olive oil and lemon cocktail), and reduce the amount of brown rice or quinoa consumed to two servings per day. I suggest you eat yams, carrots, beets, or other starchy vegetables as your main starches whenever possible. You will be enjoying an abundance of alkalizing fresh (organic) plant foods, including high quality plant-based protein.

This is a great time to juice vegetables, make green smoothies, and drink vegetable broths. These all help keep the body fortified with nutrients, while facilitating detoxification. This will be the most restrictive phase. For some people, you may want to take things deeper and really clear and restore the body. You can do the lemonade/limeade fast at this time (see lemonade fast instructions).

147

Phase 3: Adding Back and Awareness (7 – 14 days)

At this point you will be adding back the foods you eliminated during Phase 2. This can be a difficult time because you will be adding back foods that may have been causing you irritation, so take it slow. The first step is to stick with the foods on the "foods you will enjoy" list. This means you will be adding back animal foods and more grains.

Be sure the animal protein is organic. You will do this for the first four days. After the fourth, you can start to add in the other food groups we eliminated, such as dairy, gluten, sugar, and fermented foods.

However, when you add these foods, add them one at a time and journal about any symptoms you notice, such as:

- Headaches
- Sore throat
- Sinus pressure or changes with your sinuses
- Dry skin
- Moodiness
- Stomach issues
- Irregular bowel movements
- Gas
- Dry eyes
- Disrupted sleep
- Bloating
- Weight gain

As you add back food groups, keep track of symptoms so you can identify food sensitivities and understand how certain foods affect you. This will help you understand how and why you are feeling a certain way. For example, too much alcohol is known to cause hangovers. Food, especially sugars, works the same way.

If you have been doing the lemonade fast, stay with just raw salads, green smoothies, cooked vegetables (including yams), and vegetable soups, along with the suggested protein for the first 3-4 days following the lemonade fast. (You can follow the sample schedule for Phase 2 of the cleanse). Then you can reintroduce animal protein and whole grains listed on the "good food" list, following the sample schedule for Phase 3 in the basic cleanse.

Daily Stress Relief

This is one of the most important parts of your program, so please make time for it. These activities will increase endorphins in your bloodstream, which will enhance your success.

- Daily: Every morning, set the intention for your day. "I will follow my rehab program flawlessly today", "I will make someone smile today."

- Daily: Every evening write in your gratitude journal. Sit quietly and reflect on three things that you are grateful for. Write them down on paper. This quick practice can be life changing for your mindset.

- Daily: Do the Toxin Eliminator Bath. Each evening, place two cups of Epsom salts and one cup of baking soda into a tub, run the hottest water you can stand and add eight drops of lavender oil. Soak for twenty minutes and allow yourself to sweat. When you are finished bathing, wrap yourself up in towels and go under the covers and sweat some more. You should feel very relaxed and sleep soundly.

- I highly recommend you get up and move at least once a day (2 times a day is IDEAL - 1 morning, 1 sunset). This will reboot your system. Try meditation, yoga, dance, jumping on a rebounder, or taking a walk.

- Twice per week, go for a sauna

- During Phase 2, aim to do a castor oil pack each night
- At least one massage is highly recommended during your cleanse. It can be great to get one at the beginning and one towards to end, as you will see how your body has changed

Optional

Lemonade/Limeade Fast (optional in Phase 2) – Good for the following:

- Blood sugar imbalances (not diabetes)
- Candida
- Cellulite
- Skin problems
- Total internal cleansing/colon
- Liver

Optional Lemonade Cleanse – Phase 2 (2-3 days)

This fast can be quite profound. This is totally safe to do as long as you follow the instructions. The only contraindications would be pregnancy, breastfeeding, and diabetes. I suggest doing it for at least 2 days, maybe 3 days, 7 days maximum.

*If you choose to implement this, please reach out for additional support.

Shopping list for Lemonade Fast:

- Lemons (or limes)
- Cayenne pepper
- Grade B maple syrup
- Filtered or purified water
- Optional: Herbal laxative tea with senna and/or cascara

*Use organic ingredients whenever possible.

How to make your lemonade drink:
Ingredients:

*   FRESH squeezed lemon or lime juice (organic, if possible)
*   Genuine organic maple syrup, Grade B (the darker the better)
*   Cayenne pepper
*   spring or filtered water

To make a 10-ounce glass:

*   2 tablespoons fresh lemon or lime juice (absolutely no canned or frozen juice)
*   2 tablespoons grade B or C maple syrup (Don't use Grade A maple syrup or maple-flavored syrup. They are over-refined, which means that they are mostly refined sugars and lack essential minerals).
*   1/10 teaspoon cayenne pepper

Use fresh lemons or limes only, never canned or frozen juice (use organic and vine ripened when possible). Do not use Meyer lemons because they are a hybrid lemon (a cross between lemons and tangerines). Also, mix your lemonade fresh just before drinking. You can, however, squeeze your lemons in the morning and use them as needed throughout the day.

You must take a sip of the lemonade at least every 15 minutes while awake. This is very important to keep your blood sugar stable. Drink as much of this lemonade as you want, but make sure you drink at least twelve 1/4-liter (8 oz) glasses per day. Eat no other food during this cleanse but do be sure to drink plenty of purified water or herbal tea in addition to the limeade drink. The limeade contains all the vitamins and minerals you will need during the metabolic rehab.

Going off the Lemonade Fast

Your body won't be used to having solid food in it, so start with very simple foods that are easy to digest such as a protein shake or some lightly steamed veggies, salad, green smoothie, or veggie juice.

Helpful cleanse information during the Lemonade Fast:

- During the lemonade fast, stop taking all supplements
- During this fast, it is best to avoid strenuous exercise. Restorative yoga, walking, and light activity are great methods of exercises during this cleanse. If you decide to do any sort of exercise, be sure to have your lemonade/limeade drink handy.
- Listen to your body. If you feel like resting, rest. If you feel like taking a nap, nap.

Food Intolerance – Why Are We Eliminating Certain Foods?

Do you have a favorite food that you HAVE to have or can't stop eating? Do you feel tired, bloated, and drained ALL of the time? These may be signs of a food addiction or food intolerance. And if you're thinking, "Okay, so what's the big deal?" You should know it takes only ONE food to wreak havoc on your health and your ability to maintain a healthy weight, immunity, and more.

Many times, the foods we think we LOVE the most are actually the foods our bodies have a sensitivity to or intolerance to, keeping us from losing weight and making us feel tired and depressed.

When we eat a food we have an intolerance or sensitivity to, it causes an inflammatory reaction and floods our body with chemicals. And it's the chemicals our body releases that we can become addicted to and could be keeping us from losing weight, causing us to be tired and starting a cascade of other symptoms. One reason is our immune system can attack the food much like it would attack a germ, taxing your whole body and draining your energy.

Food allergies and intolerances are much more common than most people realize.

Millions of adults and children suffer from allergic reactions to food and do not know it because the symptoms can be hard to diagnose. The

152

reason a food intolerance is so difficult to identify is that there are so many different symptoms and the symptoms are different for everyone. Also, there is often a delayed reaction from eating the food, so you may eat wheat one day and feel fine, but then the next day you feel bloated and tired.

More common allergies are really more like food sensitivities and because the symptoms are bloating, poor digestion, headaches, lethargy, depression, and weight gain, most people don't think they're caused by the food they've been eating their entire lives. They just think, "There must be something wrong with me." The most common foods people have a sensitivity or intolerance to are dairy, wheat/gluten, and soy. (Gluten is the portion of the wheat that causes the problems, and it also found in other gluten grains.) These are the foods that often end up being trigger foods for people, along with sugar.

When people don't know that a food intolerance is the root cause of their health issue, they usually blame it on their slow metabolism or their bad genetics and they just live with it. Once you have eliminated these reactive foods from your life, you will be amazed at how quickly your energy and health will increase and, if needed, weight will effortlessly fall off. Your body will thank you for returning it to its natural state of radiant health.

Symptoms caused by food intolerances:

- Acne/skin breakouts

- Anxiety

- Gas/bloating

- Slow metabolism

- Depression

- Headaches

- Lethargy

- Weight gain

153

- Digestive issues
- Cravings for food
- Binge eating

Individual Issues

If you suffer from any of these issues and would like to address them during or after the 21 Days to Hormone Harmony program, please let me know. There are additional actions you can take to address these issues. This program can be a great starting point for those suffering with these conditions. However, I urge you reach out for additional help.

Candida /Yeast

Do you know what candida is? It's a clinical term for yeast and it's a sneaky little organism that can live inside your body and may be sabotaging your health, energy, and weight loss efforts.

Everyone has candida in their body. It's totally normal, and it lives in your intestines. But if you have an overgrowth, it can wreak havoc on your body and affect every area of your health.

Many people have a candida overgrowth in their bodies and don't even know it. If you've ever been on antibiotics, chances are, you ended up with a yeast infection. The reason for that is the antibiotics kill off the good bacteria in your body and allow the yeast to take over. I don't just mean a vaginal yeast infection – both men and women can have an overgrowth and it can take over lots of different parts of your body. In fact, if you have a vaginal yeast infection that means the yeast is most likely overgrown throughout your whole body.

How does this affect you? What does yeast really do to your body? It causes every health issue you have to be worse. If you have psoriasis, it will get worse. If you're depressed, you'll be more depressed. If you have headaches, they'll be worse. If you have arthritis, it will be worse. If you want to lose weight, it'll be an uphill battle. Whatever ails you will be exacerbated by the yeast overgrowth in your body. Candida isn't causing these issues, but it is making them worse.

154

So, how can you tell if you have a candida overgrowth? If you have jock itch or athlete's foot, if you get vaginal yeast infections, if you have thrush in your mouth or a white coating on your tongue, if you have a strong addiction to sugary, starchy foods or a bad sweet tooth, it's almost guaranteed that you have a candida overgrowth.

Some other symptoms include:

Chronic abdominal gas, headaches/migraines, excessive fatigue and brain fog, intense sugar and alcohol cravings, mood swings, rectal itching, itchy skin, acne, low sex drive, nail fungus, hyperactivity, anxiety or nervousness, being strongly reactive to cigarette smoke, and belly fat.

Blood Sugar Imbalance

Blood Sugar Imbalance is a condition in which your body does not handle glucose effectively. Throughout the day, blood glucose levels may fluctuate outside of the body's desired blood glucose range. Your energy can swing from being high after a meal to being low if you skip a meal. Insulin is the hormone responsible for keeping the blood sugar levels in the normal desired range. Insulin works by opening channels on cell membranes, allowing glucose to travel from the blood into body cells. During times of blood sugar imbalance, insulin can become a little out of control.

In some situations, like after a carbohydrate or sugar-rich meal, too much insulin is produced. When insulin is high, lots of cell glucose channels become open, which results in the blood glucose level dropping too low. During insulin resistance, the cell membranes have difficulty recognizing insulin and too few channels are opened. In this situation, both insulin and glucose remain high in the blood and some cells stay deficient in glucose. Cells in the pancreas secrete insulin into the blood stream. These cells can often become exhausted after long periods of producing excessive levels of insulin. Once tired, these cells can no longer produce adequate amounts of insulin to achieve perfect blood sugar balance. Low insulin production also leads to blood sugar imbalance.

Blood sugar imbalance can be a precursor to diabetes mellitus and it is therefore important to address the contributing factors before the condition develops further.

Signs your blood sugar may be out of balance:

- Cravings for sweets, sugar, or bread products (This is an almost guaranteed sign that your blood sugar is out of balance)
- Fatigue after eating a meal or a "food-coma"
- Lightheadedness if meals are missed
- Eating sweets does not relieve the cravings for sweets
- Dependence on coffee to keep yourself going or get started
- Difficulty losing weight

Hormonal, Thyroid, and Adrenal Imbalances Symptoms of female hormone imbalance:

- Acne or oily skin
- Bloating
- Bone loss
- Decreased fertility
- Depression
- Excess facial and body hair
- Hot flashes
- Heavy or painful periods
- Irregular periods
- Irritability
- Loss of muscle mass
- Loss of scalp hair
- Low libido

- Memory lapses
- Mood swings
- Nervousness
- Night sweats
- Poor concentration
- Sleep disturbances
- Tender or fibrocystic breasts
- Urinary incontinence
- Vaginal dryness
- Weight gain

Symptoms of adrenal imbalance:

- Allergies / asthma
- Sugar cravings
- Arthritis
- Sleep disturbances
- Bone loss
- Memory lapse
- Chemical sensitivities
- Morning/evening fatigue
- High blood sugar
- Increased abdominal fat

In Closing

Remember, the first 2 -3 days are usually the most challenging. It actually gets easier the longer you are on the program. Once you overcome the food addiction withdrawal, you will feel like a new person. As you stick with this program you will become more aware of your body and how food is affecting you. You will become your own detective. Having this knowledge gives you the freedom to know what, when, and how much you want to eat – based on how it makes you feel. Once you make the connection of how certain foods are affecting you, you will not miss the foods that were making you feel miserable.

I wish you great success with this program and suggest you come back to it a few times a year.

You'll find over 35 delicious recipes, including snacks and desserts, along with simple yet powerful toxin reduction strategies and daily practices, all designed to balance your hormones, boost your metabolism and help you look and feel youthful.

Download your 21 Days to Hormone Harmony Workbook (along with a bunch of other bonuses)

https://glownaturalwellness.com/hormoneharmony

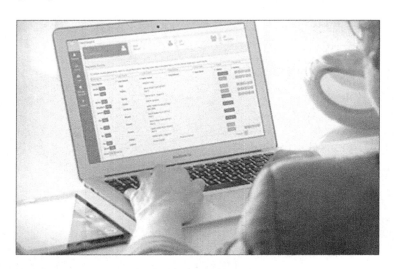

The following pages contain the meal plans, recipes, shopping guides toxin reduction practices, food prep tips, and daily protocol sheets to guide your journey.

21 Day Metabolic Rehab Meal Plan and Recipes

PHASE ONE&THREE
sample
meal plan

	BREAKFAST	LUNCH	DINNER	SNACKS & TREATS
MON	Tropical Fruit Smoothie	Adzuki Bean & Asparagus Salad	Lemony Spring Quinoa & Spinach Blueberry Salad	Crispy Chickpeas / Chopped Berries with Mint & Coconut Butter
TUES	Easy Breakfast Burrito	Leftover Lemony Spring Quinoa	Shrimp and Avocado Salad	Strawberry Mango Mint Icee / Mango Sticky Rice
WED	Creamy Rice Cereal – save leftovers for Friday	Leftover Spinach & Blueberry Salad	Curried Carrot Soup & Dandelion Greens with Ghee	Mango Sticky Rice/ Chopped Berries with Mint & Coconut Butter
THU	Red Velvet Protein Smoothie	Leftover Curried Carrot Soup & Dandelion Greens with Ghee	Spring Stir Fry	Crispy Chickpeas / Strawberries N Cream Fro-Yo
FRI	Creamy Rice Cereal	Leftover Spring Stir Fry	Artichoke & Caper "Risotto" with Radish & Carrot Salad	Cheesy Kale Chips / Strawberries N Cream Fro-Yo
SAT	Pancakes with Rhubarb Compote	Leftover Artichoke & Caper "Risotto"	Roasted Beet and Lentil Bowl	Peas with Green Goddess Dip / Strawberry Mango Mint Icee
SUN	Spring Scramble	Salmon & Endive Salad	Seasonal Vegetable Curry	Peas with Green Goddess Dip / Cheesy Kale Chips

PHASE TWO
sample
meal plan

	BREAKFAST	LUNCH	DINNER	SNACKS & TREATS
MON	Spring Greens Smoothie	Adzuki Bean & Asparagus Salad	Red Lentil & Kale Soup with Radish & Carrot Salad	Fava Bean & Pea Mash / Strawberries N Cream Fro-Yo
TUES	Red Velvet Protein Smoothie	Leftover Red Lentil & Kale Soup	Seasonal Vegetable Curry	Crispy Chickpeas/ Strawberry Mango Mint Icee
WED	Creamy Rice Cereal	Leftover Vegetable Curry	Artichoke & Caper "Risotto" with Springy Citrus Salad	Crispy Chickpeas / Mango Sticky Rice
THU	Creamy Rice Cereal	Leftover Artichoke & Caper "Risotto"	Spring Stir Fry	Fava Bean and Pea Mash/ Blueberry & Apricot Crisp
FRI	Blueberry Muesli	Leftover Spring Stir Fry	Roasted Beet & Lentil Bowl with Springy Citrus Salad	Cheesy Kale Chips/ Chocolate Avocado Chia Pudding
SAT	Berry Glowing Smoothie	Leftover Roasted Beet & Lentil Bowl	Olive and Pinenut Quinoa Salad	Cheesy Kale Chips/ Chocolate Avocado Chia Pudding
SUN	Berry Glowing Smoothie	Leftover Olive and Pinenut Quinoa	Curried Carrot Soup with Spinach & Blueberry Salad	Fava Bean and Pea Mash/ Blueberry & Apricot Crisp

phase one & three
Shopping List

Produce
2lb pre-washed spinach
2lb pre-washed arugula
6 bunches of kale
1 head endive lettuce
1 bunch Swiss chard
2 bunches dandelion greens
1 head red cabbage
4 bunches carrots
1 bunch celery
4 bunches asparagus
3 bunches radishes
2 cups snow peas
2 cups green peas
2 cups green pea pods
1 bag mung bean sprouts
4 cucumbers
1 packages of shitake mushrooms
1 shallot
1 white onion
2 red onions
1 bunch green onions
3 heads of garlic
1 fennel bulb
1 stalk lemongrass
3 avocados
5 beets
1 green apple
2 mangos
1 kiwi
1 bunch bananas
2 pints strawberries
3 pints blueberries
2 stalks rhubarb
1 bunch basil
1 bunch parsley
2 bunches cilantro
2 bunch mint
1 bunch tarragon
4 lemons
4 limes
1 ginger root

Grains, Beans and Canned Goods
2lb of quinoa
2 cups black lentils
2lb of brown rice

1 cans of adzuki beans (Eden Organics)
1 cans of white beans (Eden Organics)
Brown Rice Farina Cereal (Bob's Red Mill)
3 cans garbanzo beans
3 cans full fat coconut milk
4 cartons of vegetable broth (4 cup size)

Condiments
Sliced Almonds
Pistachios (Shelled)
Sea Salt
Pepper
Chili flakes
Turmeric
Curry Powder
Cinnamon
Vanilla
Unrefined Coconut Oil
Coconut Butter
Extra Virgin Olive Oil
Apple Cider Vinegar
Gluten Free Tamari
Almond Butter
Liquid Stevia
1 jar capers – Non-Peril
1 jar artichoke hearts packed in water
Nutritional Yeast (Bragg's)
Unsweetened coconut flakes

Meat / Dairy / Eggs / Refrigerated Section
¼ lb cooked shrimp
1 can sustainably caught salmon
1/2 dozen eggs
ghee
1 carton of unsweetened almond milk
1 bottle of unsweetened cranberry juice
Coconut Water – to have on hand to drink
Hummus

Frozen
Frozen Peas
Frozen strawberries
Frozen mango

Miscellaneous
VEGA Chocolate Protein Powder
Chia Seeds (if you can buy in bulk get 1 cup)
Hemp Seeds (if you can buy in bulk get ½ cup)

162

phase two
Shopping List

Produce

6 bunches of kale
2 bunches Swiss chard
2lbs pre-washed spinach
1lb pre-washed arugula
2 bunch carrots
1 bunch celery*
4 bunches asparagus
3 cups snow peas
1 cup green peas
1 bunch radishes
1 bag mung bean sprouts*
2 cucumbers
1 package of shitake mushrooms
2 shallots
2 red onions
2 white onions
1 stalk lemongrass
3 heads of garlic*
4 avocados
5 beets
4 pints blueberries
1 mango
2 apricots
1 bunch bananas*
1 bunch cilantro
1 bunch basil*
2 bunches mint
1 bunch parsley
6 lemons
4 limes
1 ginger root*

Grains, Beans and Canned Goods

1lb of quinoa*
2.5lbs of brown rice
1lb black lentils
1 package Gluten Free Oats (Bob's Red Mill)
Brown Rice Farina Cereal*
1 ½ cup red lentils
1 can of adzuki beans
5 cans garbanzo beans
5 cartons of vegetable broth (4 cup size)
3 cans full fat coconut milk

Condiments

Extra Virgin Olive Oil*
Coconut oil*
Coconut Butter*
Apple Cider Vinegar*
Gluten Free Tamari*
Almond Butter*
Sliced almonds*
Pine nuts
Sea Salt*
Pepper*
Chili flakes*
Curry Powder*
Turmeric*
Cinnamon*
1 jar kalamata olives, pitted
1 jar artichoke hearts
1 jar capers*
Nutritional Yeast (Bragg's)*
Liquid Stevia*
Unsweetened coconut flakes*

Meat / Dairy / Eggs / Refrigerated Section

1 carton of unsweetened almond milk
1 bottle of unsweetened cranberry juice*
Coconut Water – get extra to drink
Ghee*

Miscellaneous

VEGA chocolate protein powder*
Raw Cacao Powder
Chia Seeds*
Hemp Seeds*

Frozen

Frozen Fava beans
Frozen blueberries
Frozen strawberries*
Frozen mango*

* These are items you may already have from week one. Do a quick inventory before shopping for week two.

breakfast

Spring Greens Smoothie
[Serves 1]

INGREDIENTS
1 cup coconut water or water
1 large handful spinach
½ banana
½ cup frozen blueberries
dash of cinnamon

Blend and enjoy!

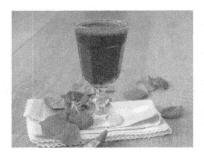

Tropical Fruit Smoothie
[Serves 1]

INGREDIENTS
½ cup unsweetened cranberry juice
½ cup fresh chopped mango
1 kiwi, skin removed
2 sprigs of mint
½ cucumber
½ cup ice

Blend and enjoy!

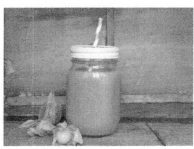

164

Red Velvet Protein Smoothie
[Serves 1]

INGREDIENTS
1 cup unsweetened almond milk
1 tablespoon almond butter
1 scoop chocolate plant protein
powder – VEGA is a great brand
1 medium beet, shredded
1 cucumber

Blend and enjoy!

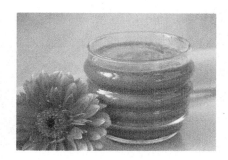

Berry Glowing Breakfast Smoothie
[Serves 1]

INGREDIENTS
1 large handful kale
1 handful spinach
½ cucumber
½ cup frozen berries – strawberry, blueberry &
  raspberry
½ cup unsweetened cranberry juice

Blend and enjoy!

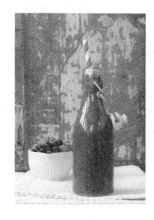

■■■ Pancakes with Rhubarb Compote
(for phase 1 and phase 3)
[Serves 2]

INGREDIENTS
3 bananas
2 eggs
½ cup almond butter
2 teaspoons cinnamon
1 teaspoon vanilla
dash of sea salt
1 tablespoon coconut oil

Combine all ingredients except oil in a blender and blend until smooth. Heat coconut oil on a skillet over medium heat. Pour ¼ cup of pancake mix on skillet and cook until lightly browned, flip over and cook until other side is lightly browned. Serve with Rhubarb compote, recipe below.

■■■ Rhubarb Compote
[Serves 2]

INGREDIENTS
2 stalks of rhubarb, chopped
1 pint of strawberries, chopped
Zest and juice of 1 lemon

Cook all ingredients over medium low heat until fruit is soft and jam like consistency about 15 minutes. Add a little water if necessary.

▪️▪️▪️ Easy Breakfast Burrito
(for phase 1 and phase 3)
[Serves 1]

INGREDIENTS
1 tablespoon coconut oil
4-5 kale leaves shredded or cut into
 ribbons
2 eggs
Lettuce leaf
4-5 basil leaves, chopped
Half an avocado
Sea salt and pepper

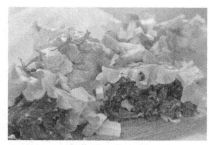

Heat oil in a pan until melted, add
kale and sauté until bright green and
a bit wilted. Crack eggs into the kale and mix to scramble the eggs. Wrap in
a lettuce leaf and top with basil and avocado. Season with salt and
pepper.

▪️▪️▪️ Spring Scramble
(for phase 1 and phase 3)
[Serves 1]

INGREDIENTS
1 tablespoon ghee
small handful of spinach
3 asparagus stalks, chopped into 1/4
 inch coins
2 eggs, beaten
½ avocado
sea salt and pepper

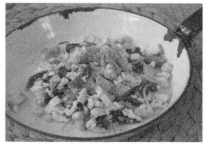

Heat ghee in a skillet, add spinach,
asparagus and sauté for 3-5 minutes.
Stir in eggs and cook for 3 more
minutes until cooked through. Top with
avocado and season with salt and pepper.

■■■ Blueberry Muesli
[Serves 1]

INGREDIENTS
½ cup gluten free rolled oats (Bob's Red Mill)
1 cup water or unsweetened coconut or almond milk
(from a carton)
2 tbsp hemp seeds (optional)
½ cup blueberries (optional)
Chopped mint

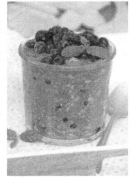

Soak all ingredients overnight and you'll have a
delicious breakfast cereal in the morning. You can
heat it up if you prefer it hot.

If you forget to soak the oats overnight, you can cook
them on the stove and then add in your fruit and
nuts.

■■■ Creamy Rice Cereal
[Serves 2]

INGREDIENTS
½ cup Brown Rice Farina Cereal
  (Bob's Red Mill)
1 cup almond milk
3/4 cup water
1 teaspoon cinnamon
1 teaspoon chia seeds
1 teaspoon sliced almonds

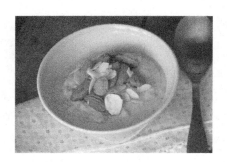

Combine all ingredients in a pot,
except almonds, and simmer for 5-8
minutes until liquid is absorbed.
Sprinkle with almonds. Enjoy!

168

lunch & dinner
■■■ Adzuki Bean and Asparagus Salad
[Serves 2]

INGREDIENTS
1 bunch thin asparagus, rough ends trimmed off
¼ cup extra virgin olive oil
Zest and juice from 1 lemon
½ bunch parsley, chopped
1 15oz can of Adzuki Beans, drained
   and rinsed (Eden Organics is great)
2 cups baby arugula
salt and pepper

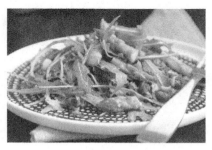

Bring a pot of water to a boil. Blanch asparagus for 5-8 minutes until tender. Remove from water and pat dry with paper towels. Chop into 1-inch pieces. Whisk the olive oil, lemon and parsley together.

In a bowl add the beans, asparagus and arugula. Toss with the dressing and season with salt and pepper.

■■■ Salmon & Endive Salad
(for phase 1 and phase 3)
[Serves 2]

INGREDIENTS
1 can of sustainably caught salmon,
   drained
½ stalk celery, diced
½ green apple, diced
1 teaspoon capers
1 tablespoon hemp seeds
2 tablespoons parsley, chopped
1 tablespoon extra virgin olive oil
salt and pepper to taste
4 -6 Endive leaves

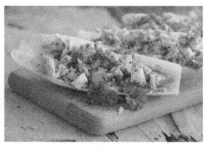

Mix all the ingredients, except endive together. Serve in endive leaves.

169

■■■ Spinach and Blueberry Salad with Lemon Basil Dressing
[Serves 4]

INGREDIENTS
8 cups baby spinach
2 pint organic blueberries
1 cup cooked quinoa or black lentils
(Trader Joe's has cooked lentils and
quinoa or you can cook your own,
recipe below.)
½ cup sliced almonds

Right before serving, mix all ingredients
in a bowl and dress.

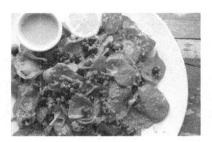

Dressing:
INGREDIENTS
6 tablespoons apple cider vinegar
1 cup extra virgin olive oil
4 cloves garlic, minced
Zest and juice of two lemons
3 tablespoons chopped basil
salt and pepper to taste

Whisk all ingredients together and dress your salad.

Quick Quinoa or Black Lentils:
INGREDIENTS
2 cups quinoa or black lentils, rinsed and soaked in lemon water for 30
 minutes
4 cups water or vegetable broth
Dash of salt

Combine all the ingredients in a pot and bring to a boil over medium heat.
Reduce to a simmer, cover and cook until water is absorbed, 15 – 20
minutes.

Spring Stir-Fry
[Serves 2]

INGREDIENTS
Rice:
1 1/2 cup brown rice
3 cups water or veggie broth
1 garlic clove minced

Spicy Lemongrass and Garlic Sauce:
½ cup vegetable broth
½ cup Gluten Free Tamari
1 teaspoon chili flakes (less or more depending on
how much heat you like)
2 clove minced garlic
1 teaspoon minced fresh lemongrass
juice of 1 lime

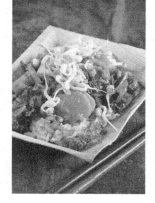

Stir-Fry:
2 tablespoons coconut oil
1 small white onion
2 cloves of garlic minced
2 teaspoons ginger minced
1 package of Enoki or Shitake Mushrooms
½ cup snow peas
½ bunch of asparagus, cut into 1/2" pieces
2 carrots, cut into ½" pieces
½ bunch kale, cut into ribbons
1 handful mung bean sprouts

Mix the rice, garlic and broth in a pot over high heat. When the broth comes
to a boil, turn heat down to a simmer and cover. Cook until all the liquid has
been soaked in the rice about 45 minutes.

In a small saucepan combine all the ingredients for the spicy lemongrass
sauce and simmer for 5 minutes to let the flavors meld. Remove from heat.

In a wok or large pan with sides, heat coconut oil and add garlic, ginger
and onions. Let simmer until brown. Add a little more oil if needed and toss in
all of your veggies (except the sprouts). Give them a good mix and cover
your pan so the veggies can steam. Steam for 5-10 minutes depending on
how "al dente" you want your veggies.

Scoop a large spoonful of rice into a bowl; add a generous helping of
veggies, a spoonful of spicy lemongrass sauce and then top with sprouts.

■■■ Lemony Spring Quinoa
[Serves 4]

INGREDIENTS
1 cup quinoa, rinsed and soaked for 20 minutes
2 cups vegetable broth
4 cloves of garlic minced
1 small red onion, sliced
1lb baby arugula
1 15oz can of white or garbanzo beans
  (Eden Organics is a great brand)
1 small bunch of radishes, sliced
½ cup fresh peas (can also use frozen
but defrost them first)
1 carrot, grated
1 bunch of mint, cut into ribbons
½ cup pistachios
zest and juice of one lemon
¼ cup extra virgin olive oil

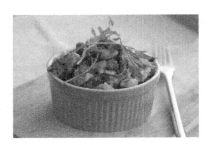

In a pot, combine quinoa, vegetable broth, garlic and red onion. Cook on medium heat for 15 – 20 minutes until liquid is absorbed. Stir in the rest of the ingredients and season with salt and pepper.

■■■ Shrimp and Avocado Salad
(for phase 1 and phase 3)

[Serves 1]

INGREDIENTS
¼ lb cooked shrimp (save time by buying
  fresh or frozen cooked shrimp)
2 cups spinach or arugula
¼ cup shredded red cabbage
1/2 avocado, sliced
Juice from one lime
2 tablespoons olive oil

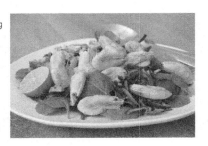

Serve shrimp on the bed of greens, avocado, cabbage and dress with olive oil and lime juice.

Dandelion Greens with Ghee

[Serves 4]

INGREDIENTS
2 bunches dandelion greens, cut into
 strips
¼ cup ghee, melted
½ cup nutritional yeast
salt and pepper

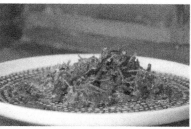

Cook dandelion greens in salted
boiling water for 15 minutes, drain and
squeeze out excess water. Coarsely
chop and place in your serving dish. Drizzled melted ghee on the greens
and then toss with nutritional yeast, salt and pepper.

Olive and Pinenut Quinoa Salad

[Serves 4]

INGREDIENTS
1 cup quinoa, rinsed and soaked for 20
 minutes
2 cups vegetable broth
¼ cup pitted kalamata olives, chopped
½ cup toasted pine nuts
2 cups baby spinach
2 tablespoons lemon juice
¼ cup extra virgin olive oil
salt and pepper to taste

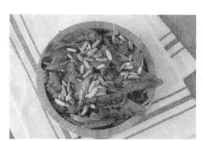

In a pot, combine quinoa and vegetable broth. Cook on medium heat
covered for 15 – 20 minutes until liquid is absorbed. Stir in the rest of the
ingredients and season with salt and pepper.

▪▪▪ Springy Salad with Citrus Dressing

[Serves 4]

INGREDIENTS
1 head of kale, cut into small ribbons
1 small bunch of red radishes, sliced
1 cup snow peas
2 carrots, diced
1/2 small red onion, sliced
1 avocado, chopped
2 tablespoons hemp seeds
1 can of garbanzo beans drained
and rinsed

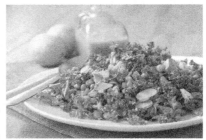

Combine all ingredients in a large
bowl. Dress only what you will eat with
the dressing below.

Dressing:
INGREDIENTS
¼ cup fresh squeezed lemon juice
2 tablespoons apple cider vinegar
2/3 cup extra virgin olive oil
2 tablespoons garlic, chopped
1 teaspoon pepper
sea salt

Whisk all ingredients together and season with salt. Pour enough onto salad
to coat all the veggies.

Artichoke and Caper "Risotto"

[Serves 4]

INGREDIENTS
2 cups vegetable broth
1 cup short grain brown rice
2 tablespoons ghee
1 shallot, thinly sliced
3 cloves garlic, minced
1 bunch Swiss chard, cut into ribbons
1 jar of artichoke hearts, drained
2 tablespoon capers
1 handful chopped parsley
salt and pepper

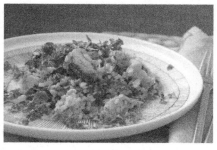

Combine the vegetable broth and rice in a small pot over high heat. When the broth comes to a boil, turn heat down to a simmer and cover. Cook until all the liquid has been soaked in the rice about 45 minutes.

While rice cooks, heat 2 tablespoons of ghee in a sauté pan and cook shallots until melted, about 8 minutes. Add garlic and swiss chard and cook for 5 more minutes. Add artichokes and capers and cook for 2 more minutes.

Combine the rice, Swiss chard mixture and parsley in a bowl. Season with salt and pepper.

For added protein you can add a can of garbanzo beans.

■■■ Curried Carrot Soup

[Serves 4]

INGREDIENTS
1 tablespoon ghee
1 ½" piece of ginger, sliced and crushed
4 cloves garlic, minced
Zest and juice of one lime
2 teaspoons curry powder
1 teaspoon turmeric
3 cups carrots cut into 1" pieces
1 15oz can of full fat coconut milk (I
  recommend Native Forest brand)
2 cups water
½ bunch cilantro, chopped

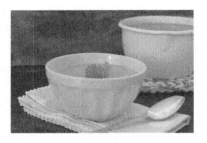

Heat ghee in a large saucepan over medium heat. Add ginger, garlic, and lime zest and cook until slightly browned, about 3-4 minutes. Add curry and turmeric and cook until fragrant - about 1 minute. Add carrots, coconut milk and water. Bring to a boil, reduce to low and simmer, covered, for 15 minutes. Turn off heat and leave on stove for ½ hour to allow flavors to meld.

Puree soup in blender or food processor. Garnish with chopped cilantro, lime juice and enjoy!

Seasonal Vegetable Curry

[Serves 4]

INGREDIENTS
2 tablespoons coconut oil
1 onion, peeled and diced
1 tbsp. curry powder
2 carrots, peeled and diced
½ cup snow peas
1 bunch asparagus
2 cups garbanzo beans, cooked or
  canned
1 15oz can of unsweetened
  coconut milk (I recommend Native
  Forest brand)
4 cups vegetable broth
2 bunches of any type of greens,
washed and cut (kale, bok choy, escarole, collards, turnip greens, etc.)
Salt and pepper to taste
Fresh cilantro for garnish

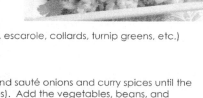

In a large pot heat coconut oil and sauté onions and curry spices until the
onions are soft (about 6-8 minutes). Add the vegetables, beans, and
coconut milk. Bring to simmer and add the vegetable broth. Simmer until
the veggies are tender (about 15 minutes). Add the greens, then season
with salt and pepper.

Serve with brown rice. Garnish with cilantro.

▬▬▬ Roasted Beet and Lentil Bowl with Avocado Cilantro Sauce

[Serves 4]

INGREDIENTS
1 cup black lentils, rinsed
2 cups water or vegetable broth
4 medium beets, roasted (see notes)
1 bunch asparagus, chopped into bite sized pieces
1 large avocado
½ cup cilantro leaves
1 garlic clove
2 teaspoons lime juice (1 lime)
salt and pepper to taste
2 tablespoons water or unsweetened almond milk
2 teaspoons extra virgin olive oil

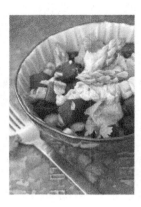

Pre-heat oven to 400°

Combine the lentils and water or broth in a pot over medium high heat and cook until water is absorbed and lentils are tender – about 15 minutes.

Wash and peel the beets. Wrap in foil and roast for 45 minutes until tender. Brush the asparagus with olive oil and add to the baking sheet with the beets for the last 10 minutes of cook time.

In a blender, combine the avocado, cilantro, garlic, lime juice, salt and pepper and blend. Add water slowly until you have a sauce consistency. Divide the lentils into 2 bowls, top with chopped asparagus, beets and drizzle with avocado sauce.

Note: all of this can be made in advance and stored in the fridge for 4 days. I recommend making extra of everything to save time and energy.

178

Red Lentil and Kale Soup
[Serves 4]

INGREDIENTS
1 tablespoon coconut oil
1 medium onion, finely chopped
4 garlic cloves, minced
2 large carrots, chopped
2 stalks of celery, chopped
1 bunch of kale, cut into ribbons
6 cups of vegetable broth
1 ½ cup red lentils, rinsed
salt and pepper to taste

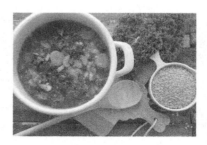

Heat the oil in a large pot over medium heat. Add the onion and sauté until translucent – 3-5 minutes. Add the garlic, carrots, celery and kale and sauté for 2-3 minutes. Add the broth, lentils, salt and pepper. Cook on medium-low heat until lentils are tender, 20 minutes.

Radish and Carrot Ribbon Salad
[Serves 4]

INGREDIENTS
2 bunches radishes, thinly sliced
6 carrots, thinly sliced into ribbons (a vegetable peeler works great)
1 fennel, thinly sliced
Small handful chopped parsley

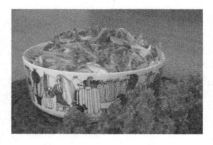

Dressing
INGREDIENTS
3 tablespoons apple cider vinegar
1 tablespoon lime juice
½ cup extra virgin olive oil
1 garlic clove, minced

Mix ingredients and toss with the salad dressing.

snacks

Fava Bean, Pea and Mint Mash
[Serves 4]

INGREDIENTS
1 cup fava beans (buy frozen and thaw)
1 cup baby peas (buy frozen and thaw)
Zest and juice from one lemon
¼ cup extra virgin olive oil
2 tablespoons mint, chopped
Salt and pepper to taste
Carrots or celery to eat the mash with

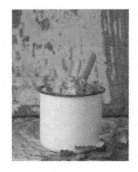

Add all the ingredients to a food processor and
process until mashed but still a few whole pieces in it.

Chopped Berries with Mint and Coconut Butter
[Serves 1]

INGREDIENTS
1 cup of mixed berries – blueberries,
strawberries and raspberries
2 tablespoons coconut butter, melted
1 tablespoon chopped mint

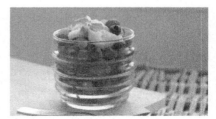

Drizzle the melted coconut butter on
the berries and sprinkle with mint.

Cheesy Kale Chips
[Serves 2]

INGREDIENTS
2 heads of kale torn into large pieces
4 teaspoons extra virgin olive oil
2 tablespoon nutritional yeast
sea salt and pepper

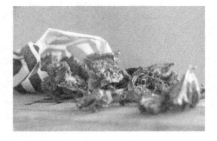

Toss kale with oil and season with
nutritional yeast and sea salt. Bake for
15 - 20 minutes at 300° or until crispy –
being careful not to burn.

treats

Mango Sticky Rice
[Serves 2]

INGREDIENTS
3/4 cup brown rice
1 15oz can of full fat coconut milk (I
  recommend Native Forest brand)
2-3 drops stevia
1 mango, cut into slices

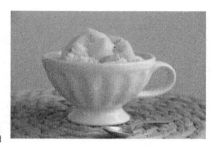

Cook rice and coconut milk together in
a pan over medium low heat until liquid
is absorbed, about 15 – 20 minutes. Stir in stevia and top with mango.

Strawberry Mango Mint Icee
[Serves 1]

INGREDIENTS
1/2 cup frozen strawberries
½ cup frozen mango
1 tablespoon chopped mint
1 teaspoon lime juice
1 tablespoon unsweetened coconut

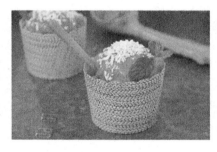

Blend strawberries, mint and lime juice.
Top with coconut.

Chocolate Avocado Chia Pudding
[Serves 2]

INGREDIENTS
1 cup unsweetened almond milk (in a
  carton, not canned)
¼ cup chia seeds
2 avocados
½ cup cacao powder
2-3 drops of stevia

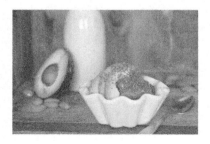

Mix all ingredients in a blender and
refrigerate for 3-4 hours or overnight.

181

■■■ Blueberry& Apricot Crisp
[Serves 2]

INGREDIENTS
2 tablespoons melted coconut butter
1 pint blueberries
2 fresh apricots, pits removed and
  chopped
1 cup gluten free oats (Bob's Red Mill is
  great)
¼ sliced almonds
2 teaspoons cinnamon
1 tablespoon coconut oil, melted

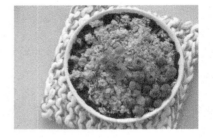

Heat oven to 375°.

Coat 2 ramekins or small oven proof bowls with coconut butter. Mix blueberries and apricots together and divide into ramekins. Mix oatmeal, almonds, cinnamon and coconut oil together and top the fruit.

Cook crisps for 15 – 20 minutes until slightly brown and bubbly.

■■■ Strawberries and Cream Fro-Yo
[Serves 2]

INGREDIENTS
2 frozen bananas
1 cup frozen strawberries
¼ cup unsweetened almond milk
1 tablespoon hemp seeds

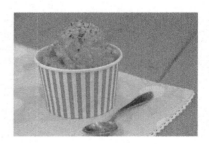

Place bananas and strawberries into your blender and blend while slowly adding the almond milk until you have the consistency of frozen yogurt. You may not need to use all ¼ cup of almond milk. Top with hemp seeds.

Toxin reduction tips and tools

Water – Be sure the number of ounces of water you drink per day is equal to at least half of your body weight. (i.e. 150 lbs. body weight = 75 oz. water per day). In the autumn and winter, it can be especially helpful and cleansing to drink warm water.

Lemon Water – This is a gentle yet effective way to support and cleanse the liver, kidneys, and colon, and help alkalize the body. It assists in breaking up mucus and provides energy via enzymes, vitamin C, potassium, and trace minerals. Please use fresh, ripe lemons, not prepared lemon juice. Make lemon water simply by squeezing the juice of ½ a lemon into a glass of water.

Body Brushing – This is one of best ways to stimulate the lymphatic system. This is beneficial because it assists the lymph nodes in keeping blood and other vital tissues detoxified. It is energizing, assists in breaking up cellulite, removes dead skin, stimulates circulation, and strengthens the immune system. To do this, you will need a natural bristle brush, which can be purchased at most health food stores or pharmacies. Start at your feet and work up the body in long strokes towards your heart. Be sure to cover the whole body, but skip the face and the breasts. Do not feel like you need to spend a tremendous amount of time on this, 2–3 minutes prior to your shower is fine.

Toxin Elimination Bath – Each evening, place 2 cups of Epsom salts and one cup of baking soda in the tub, run the hottest water you can stand, and add 8 drops lavender oil. Soak for 20 minutes and allow yourself to sweat. When you are finished bathing, wrap yourself up in towels, go under the covers, and sweat some more. You should feel very relaxed and sleep soundly.

Exercise – Moving will be a key component to your cleanse. Tune into to what kind of exercise feels appropriate, rather than just doing what you usually do or what you think you should do. Walking, yoga, swimming, tai chi, hiking, biking, and strength training are all great ways to get moving. A powerful exercise for removing toxins is using a mini-trampoline or rebounder to help enhance you lymphatic system. This is called Lymphasizing, see the end of this document for more details.

Fiber – Getting additional fiber as we cleanse is vital to supporting the colon in its role of toxin elimination. In addition to lots of fresh vegetables, ground flax seeds and chia seeds are recommended. You should be eliminating at least 2 times per day.

Castor oil packs – This can be a self-administered and inexpensive way to nurture and support the liver while you cleanse. It is incredibly healing and relaxing. Castor oil is said to be able to penetrate deeply – as much as 4 inches – into the body. These packs can be used to stimulate and detox the liver and gall bladder.

Directions:

- You will need 100% pure, cold-pressed castor oil, an old T-shirt, and a hot water bottle (or heating pad)
- Put on an old T-shirt, so you don't get the oil on your nice clothing
- Rub castor oil on your abdomen, being sure to cover the area where your liver is
- Lie down on you back, and place the hot water bottle or heating pad on your abdomen, on top of your shirt, for one hour
- Alternatively, you can rub the castor oil on your back, being sure to cover the area where your liver is. Then with your T-shirt on, lay on top of the heating pad or hot water bottle.

This is a safe regimen to continue throughout the spring season, especially if you suffer from liver-based symptoms like eye problems, PMS, pre-menopausal symptoms and menopausal irritability, mood swings, bloating, tender breasts, hot flashes, anxiety, migraines, skin rashes and break-outs, angry outbursts, or tension between the shoulders.

Many people report a remarkable sense of well-being and tranquility while applying the castor oil pack. Because the emotion of anger is closely tied to the liver, you may experience angry feelings resurfacing. Stay with your feelings and try to channel them constructively. You may try to transform this anger into forgiveness - first for yourself and then for others.

■■■ Metabolic Meditations

Chewing Meditation

As you enjoy a meal, take the time to chew each bite fully, 30–50 chews per bite. The objective is to liquefy your food. Focus on the taste and texture and how they might change and sweeten the longer you chew. Go slowly and really savor the experience. The added benefit of this meditation is improved digestion. Don't forget to chew your soups and smoothies!

Savoring Simplicity

This is a bit more general, but focuses on tuning into a single food or a simple dish. Enjoy the sweet crunch of a carrot, the juicy delight of a strawberry. Tune into the complexity of these seemingly simple foods. Spend at least a full five minutes with each simple food.

Breathing Meditation

This is a wonderful one that will calm and center you in any situation. It can also be used when you feel overwhelmed by a craving. Very often the craving will pass by the end of 10–20 breaths.

To practice: Close your eyes, place your hands on your belly and just tune into the sensations around the inhale and the exhale. Gradually begin to deepen the breath, taking 10–20 slow deep conscious breaths deeply into and out of the belly. Do this meditation often.

Visualization

Now is a wonderful time to put attention on what you would like to bring into your life and one of the most powerful tools you can use is images. By creating images in your mind and connecting emotionally with these images, you begin to send the message to the universe that this is what you want. If creating images in your mind is difficult, cut pictures out of magazines or other media that represent your goals and dreams. This is a powerful tool, so really take the time to work on what you DO want. When visualizing, stay with your image and the feelings it evokes for a good 3-5 minutes.

Gratitude Meditation

So simple yet immensely powerful, the gratitude meditation is highly recommended. It is especially important if you often find yourself spiraling down the hole of negative thinking and negative manifestations in your life.

This can be done anytime, but it can be particularly good first thing in the morning or before going to bed. Sit quietly with your eyes closed and meditate on all that is good in your life. If you are having trouble finding something good, simply feel gratitude for the gift of breath and a healthy body. Your objects of gratitude can be as big or as small as you want. You may choose to write down these items after or before meditating on them. Do this for as long as you want. You can also do this while walking in nature.

Walking Meditation

With walking meditation, the intention is on fully taking in the smells, the sights, the sounds and the sensations of your walking experience. Try to put your attention on only one thing or one sensory organ at a time. Take the time to drop in and just allow any thoughts outside your present experience to fall by the wayside. This can be a great meditation if you have trouble sitting still.

▰▰▰ Breathing

Two wonderful breathing techniques for cleansing:

Sounding Breath is done lying on the ground in the corpse pose, letting all your limbs relax. Exhale completely and then slowly draw in your breath through the nose. As you inhale, feel how your lungs and abdomen fill up. As you exhale, contract your throat to make a slight hissing sound and completely exhale and empty your lungs. Let your breath be long and slow.

Sitting Breath is done while sitting, so it can be done at any point. Exhale with a deep sigh in order to reset your diaphragm. Then breathe slowly through your nose for a count of 7, and hold your breath for a count of 7. Then for another count of 7, exhale through your nose. Repeat this three times, and this will help calm your spirit and relax your nerves.

The benefits of doing Pranayama (breathing exercises) every morning (or evening) for 20 to 25 minutes include:

- Increases lung capacity and improves breathing efficiency
- Improves circulation, normalizes blood pressure and improves cardiovascular efficiency
- Boosts the immune system and enhances immunity
- Increases energy levels and gives lots of positive energy
- Strengthens and tones the nervous system
- Combats anxiety and depression and improves sleep
- Improves digestion and excretory functions
- Provides massage to the internal organs, stimulates the glands and enhances endocrine functions,
- Normalizes body weight and provides great conditioning for weight loss

■■■ Power of Breathing

Undoubtedly, the most important component to human health and vitality is oxygen. In fact, human life would not be possible without it. Oxygen produces ATP (adrenosine triphosphate) and without ATP, our bodies would immediately shut down. When a person breathes, there is an exchange of carbon dioxide and oxygen. The oxygen, which is taken in by the body from the atmosphere around us, is picked up by the hemoglobin in the blood and distributed to all of the body's trillions of cells where it is then used to fuel the cells and release energy (ATP).

In addition, the makeup of the human body is largely composed of the element oxygen, especially factoring in that water is composed of 33% oxygen.

188

It's clear that optimal oxygenation of your cells through proper nutrition, fluid intake, exercise, and stress management is absolutely necessary in order to maintain your health and create a vital life.

Improper breathing is a common cause of ill health. If I had to limit my advice on healthier living to just one tip, it would be simply to learn how to breathe correctly. There is no single more powerful – nor simpler - daily practice to further your health and wellbeing than breath work.

■■■ Power of Lymphasizing - The Benefits of Rebounding

* The vertical use of acceleration, deceleration, and gravity provide the ideal conditions for cleansing cells

* Rebounding is a true cellular exercise. It builds physical cellular strength by challenging the structure of each cell. This strengthening of the cells helps to protect against degenerative disease.

* It leads to improved posture, increased vascularity, better muscle tone, enhanced timing, sharper vision, greater coordination, better balance, more rhythm, and elevated energy levels

* By working against the constant gravitational pressure while bouncing, you resist the earth's pull. Gravity becomes a force for the good of your entire body.

* Rebounding will let you improve the working of your heart muscle by improving the tine and quality of the muscle itself and by increasing the coordination of the fibers as they wring blood out of the heart during each beat

* It provides the stimulus for a free-flowing lymphatic drainage system, which helps rid your body of toxins, cancer cells, wastes, trapped protein, bacteria viruses, and other waste the cells cast off

* When you are rebounding, you are flooding the cells with oxygen. This enables them to convert glucose into ATP and also into glycogen. Thus, rebounding can actually increase your ability to convert

189

glucose into glycogen. Further, it may be possible to train your body (through consistent lymphasizing) to store this glycogen and have it released when you need it for a sudden burst of energy.

Something To Think About - The G-force (gravity) at the top of the bounce is eliminated and the body becomes weightless for a fraction of a second. At the bottom of the bounce, the G-force suddenly doubles over what is ordinary gravity on earth, and internal organs are put under pressure. Their cellular stimulation is increased accordingly so waste materials within cells get squeezed out. The lymphatics carry the waste away to be disposed of through the urinary tract and other excretory mechanism.

I have found the power of vital breathing and lymphasizing to be a master principle of a vital life.

Food Preparation and Cooking Tips

■■■ I know how hard it can be to follow a meal plan when you are a busy mom, so I put together some tips and tricks to save you time and frustration.

■■■ Food Preparation

- Prepare vegetables in advance. Cut up enough veggies to last a few days, both for snacking and cooking.

- Make extra brown rice – cook the whole bag if you can. This way it is ready and you just need to reheat as needed.

- Use organic frozen vegetables and fruit

- Soak rice, beans, and nuts overnight to remove to make them easier to digest. If using canned beans rinse well, then soak for 2 hours.

- Double one of the smoothie recipes in the morning and have it as a snack

- Use canned or bagged wild Alaskan canned salmon (but not during Phase 2)

■■■ Cooking Tips & Techniques

- Vegetables: Steam, water sauté, or roast your vegetables

- Spice up your food – add herbs and spices to your cooking. Adding fresh rosemary, chopped cilantro, chives, or parsley helps enhance the flavor and reduces the need to add fat. You can also add fresh crushed garlic to your vegetables.

- Roast a bulb of garlic and use it like you would butter. (Try it, it works!).

- When cooking fish or chicken, grill or broil and season with herbs

- Use aromatics – scallions, bulb onions, ginger, garlic and lemongrass. They add flavor and aroma to foods.

- Choose vegetables from all categories – eat the ones you like and try something new

- Use extra virgin olive oil or avocado oil and salt and pepper for dressings whenever possible

- For cooking, use coconut oil, ghee, or avocado oil

Daily Protocol

■■■Phase 1 Daily Protocol

Start reducing sugars and stimulants. All animal protein should be organic. Feel free to add additional animal protein to recipes if you desire. Always be sure that you know what your meals and snacks are going to be in advance. You can follow the meal plan in the recipe book or you can freestyle it. (Freestyle: Eat foods from the approved lists – but not necessarily in the recipes.

Upon Arising

- Stretch and practice deep breathing to replenish yourself
- Hydrate with 16 oz purified water with juice of ½ lemon
- Dry brush or hot towel scrub
- Exercise in whatever way feels appropriate
- Take a probiotic and Vitamin C or Ester C
- Set your intention for the day

Breakfast

- Cup of green tea (limit to two cups per day, if caffeinated)
- Breakfast option of your choice

Mid-morning

- Hydrate
- Take a standing forward bend or walk break
- Practice one Metabolic Meditation
- Smoothie or snack of your choice

Lunch

- Hydrate with purified water with juice of ½ lemon
- Optional: Herbal tea (detox blend, nettle, or dandelion)
- Lunch option of your choice

Afternoon

- Hydrate
- Snack option of your choice
- Detox tea or green tea

Before Dinner

- Hydrate with purified water with juice of ½ lemon
- Move your body for 10 minutes

Dinner

- Dinner option of your choice

Before Bed

- Toxin Eliminator Bath
- Take 2 tbsp. ground flax or chia seeds in 6 oz. water to help stimulate morning elimination. (Only recommended if you are experiencing constipation.)
- Gratitude – for 2 minutes, name all the things you are grateful for
- Journal about your energy level/notes

194

▬■▬ Phase 2 Daily Protocol
No animal protein, deeper cleansing, metabolic support

Upon Arising

- Stretch, sigh, deep breathing, *Replenish* yourself
- Hydrate with purified water with juice of ½ lemon
- Drink the lemon and olive oil cocktail (1 tablespoon of organic extra virgin olive oil and half a squeezed lemon)
- Dry brush or hot towel scrub
- Exercise in whatever way that feels appropriate
- Take a probiotic and Vitamin C or Ester C
- Set your intention for the day

Breakfast

- Green tea (limit two cups per day, if caffeinated)
- Breakfast option of your choice

Mid-morning

- Hydrate with purified water with juice of ½ lemon
- Take a standing forward bend break if at work
- Practice one Metabolic Meditation
- Smoothie or snack of your choice

Lunch

- Lunch option of your choice
- Optional: detox tea

Afternoon

- Hydrate
- Smoothie or snack of your choice
- Detox tea

Before Dinner

- Hydrate with purified water with juice of ½ lemon
- Move your body for 10 minutes

Dinner (remember no nightshades or corn)

- Dinner option of your choice

Before Bed

- Toxin Eliminator Bath
- Castor oil pack
- Take 2 tbsp. ground flax or chia seeds in 6 oz. water to help stimulate morning elimination. (Only recommended if you are experiencing constipation.).
- Gratitude – for 2 minutes, name all the things you are grateful for
- Journal about your energy level/notes

■■■ Phase 3 Daily Protocol

Start adding back animal proteins, gluten free grains, and organic diary

Upon Arising

- Stretch, sigh, deep breathing, *Replenish* yourself
- Hydrate with purified water with juice of ½ lemon
- Dry brush or hot towel scrub
- Exercise in whatever way that feels appropriate
- Take probiotic and Vitamin C or Ester C

Breakfast

- Green tea (limit two cups per day, if caffeinated)
- Breakfast option of your choice

Mid-morning

- Hydrate
- Take a stretch break or go for a walk
- Practice one Metabolic Meditation
- Smoothie or snack of your choice

Lunch

- Lunch option of your choice
- Optional: detox tea

Afternoon

- Hydrate
- Smoothie or snack of your choice
- Optional: detox tea

Before Dinner

- Hydrate
- Move your body for 10 minutes

Dinner

- Dinner option of your choice

Before Bed

- Toxin Eliminator Bath
- Take 2 tbsp. ground flax or chia seeds in 6 oz. water to help stimulate morning elimination. (Only recommended if you are experiencing constipation.).
- Gratitude – for 2 minutes, name all the things you are grateful for
- Journal about your day, energy levels, feelings

Made in the USA
Las Vegas, NV
17 April 2023